The
AIDS
Epidemic

The
AIDS
Epidemic

Edited by
Kevin M. Cahill, M.D.

St. Martin's Press   NEW YORK

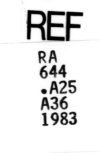
THE AIDS EPIDEMIC. Copyright © 1983 by Kevin M. Cahill, M.D.
All rights reserved. Printed in the United States of America. No part
of this book may be used or reproduced in any manner whatsoever
without written permission except in the case of brief quotations
embodied in critical articles or reviews. For information, address St.
Martin's Press, 175 Fifth Avenue, New York, N.Y. 10010.

Library of Congress Cataloging in Publication Data
Main entry under title:

The AIDS Epidemic.

    1. Acquired immune deficiency syndrome.   2. Epidemics—
United States.   I. Cahill, Kevin M.   II. Title: The AIDS
Epidemic.   [DNLM: 1. Acquired immunodeficiency
syndrome—Occurrence—United States. WD 308 A288]
RA644.A25A36   1983   616.9   83-10909
ISBN 0-312-01498-8
ISBN 0-312-01499-6 (pbk.)

10 9 8 7 6 5 4 3 2

For
Tino and Carole,
whose sensitivity matches
the complexity of this issue

Contents

II. IMMUNOLOGY

III. THE CLINICAL PICTURE

IV. IMPLICATIONS

V. THE FUTURE

Acknowledgments

The symposium that led to this book was made possible by generous grants from the Robert and Marillyn Wilson Foundation, Leonard Bernstein, the Jack Natkin Memorial Fund, and the Louis Russek Fund. Harry Kraut, Tom Steele, Charles Ortleb, and Don Armstrong helped arrange the program. I am grateful to the many people at Lenox Hill Hospital who assisted on the day of the symposium. Bill Hanlon and Michael Denneny assisted me in editing the text and Michael coordinated the book's publication at St. Martin's Press.

Invocation

Terence Cardinal Cooke

Mr. Mayor, Doctor Cahill, my friends of the medical community:

I salute each of you as we come together from all over the United States on this Sunday in spring here at Lenox Hill Hospital in New York City.

You represent many different professions within the health care community. There are here today, I understand, doctors, nurses, scientists, researchers, technicians and technologists, and many other dedicated people. You have assembled because of your concern about a major epidemic in our country that is affecting an ever-growing number of people and that has resulted already in the loss of so many lives. I support you in your daily, courageous efforts in facing this danger and in meeting this challenge.

You are here also because you are convinced that individually and collectively you have God-given powers to strengthen your brothers and sisters and to heal them. You know from experience that in teamwork and cooperation there is solid hope in finding answers to perplexing questions. This spirit of teamwork must go beyond the medical community and involve people of religious, private, and governmental sectors in making sure that this crisis becomes an opportunity to serve. In areas of research especially, in the pooling of information and knowledge, we can penetrate unknown boundaries and arrive at solutions to human problems which only seem insoluble.

You are here above all else because you are loving, caring people. Each person's pain is pain to you; each person's joy is your own. You understand the elements of the AIDS epidemic in terms of the pain and the anxiety and the fear of the individual human being—the patient—who is suffering. And you will use your skills and the scientific data which you share today to help that person.

I am one with you in your concern, and I rejoice that you are people of hope. We represent many different faiths and philosophies of life. I invite you to pray with me as we begin this important day.

Heavenly Father, eternal Spirit of Wisdom and Healing, we acknowledge Your presence among us, and we thank You for the powers which You have given us, especially the power of healing.

Lord, we pray for our brothers and sisters who are suffering from the Acquired Immune Deficiency Syndrome and for their families and friends. We ask You to inspire the members of the medical profession who are striving to strengthen and support and heal them.

Lord, as we face this crisis together, make us instruments of Your peace.

Heal our divisions and deepen our unity.

Renew our hope, and bring a sense of joy into our lives and the lives of those we serve.

Lord, replace the anxiety within us with a quiet confidence.

Replace the tension within us with a holy relaxation.

Replace the turbulence within us with a sacred calm.

Replace the coldness within us with a loving warmth.

Father, we are united in this prayer and in a spirit of faith, of hope, and of love. We ask You to assist and bless us always in our work to help our brothers and sisters in Your one human family.

Amen.

Welcome

Mayor Edward I. Koch

It is my pleasure to welcome so many physicians, scientists, and other health workers to this national gathering on the steadily escalating AIDS crisis. I welcome also the families and friends of AIDS victims. With them I share the hope and the prayer that from gatherings such as this remarkable symposium will emerge a solution to the most frightening epidemic we have faced in recent years.

New Yorkers have an almost legendary ability to handle crises. But this crisis is obviously different in kind from strikes, and blackouts, and blizzards. It's killing people and we don't know what's causing it or how to stop it.

I do not make it a habit to indulge in false modesty about this city's resources or the talents of its citizens. We have some of the finest and most respected health care and research institutions in the world and we have people working in them who, in my opinion, are second to none for dedication and intelligence. But let me tell you something. We need help in this crisis, plenty of help. Not just financial help but the help of your hands, and your minds, and your determination. That is why it is so gratifying to note the presence here today of representatives from Boston, Atlanta, Dallas, Houston, Los Angeles, San Francisco, Vancouver, Miami, Oklahoma, and elsewhere.

At present, New York bears the greatest burden of this disease. We have the unenviable record of more cases, and more fatalities, from AIDS than any other metropolitan center in the world. Still, this disease—if it is anything like other epidemics in history—will not stay confined to one group or one geographical location. It has already shown a predilection for several diverse populations.

This symposium and the resultant book bring together some of the best medical talent, both scientific and clinical, in the country. You all have the same aim: to find out what this terrible disease is that is destroying young lives and sowing such fear in parts of our community.

I have committed my administration to this vital struggle. Dr. David Sencer, my Commissioner of Health and a nationally known public health expert, is coordinating the city's response. I know you share that commitment. Together, we shall discover the cause of this deadly epidemic and stop it.

We meet under the chairmanship of Dr. Kevin M. Cahill, senior member of the New York City Board of Health, a friend, and one whose counsel and skills are always valued by myself and many others but especially in a time of medical crisis.

I salute you all for your dedication and wish you well in your deliberations.

Preface:
The Evolution of an Epidemic

Kevin M. Cahill, M.D.

Several years ago, healthy young men began to die in large numbers from an unknown disease. As so often happens in the history of medicine, the early cases were considered isolated extremes in the normal spectrum of any illness and there was, in retrospect, an inadequate appreciation by the health professions of a growing disaster. Slowly, but inexorably, the numbers afflicted grew until this insidious disease exploded into a frightening epidemic.

Persons who had been previously well developed rare tumors and unusual systemic infections. Studies indicated that these patients had suddenly and inexplicably lost their normal immunity to disease. They had an illness for which modern medicine had no name and, in our ignorance, we called it Acquired Immune Deficiency Syndrome—or AIDS.

More and more cases have been recognized since AIDS was first seen in 1979–80. At first, most of the victims were homosexual men in New York City and California, but soon heterosexual Haitians and drug addicts were diagnosed. Then blood recipients, particularly hemophiliacs, fell before this new, puzzling, and deadly epidemic. Within eighteen months over a thousand cases were reported in the United States and Europe.

There were many questions and few answers. Concern led to fear and mushroomed into panic. There were demands for drastic action, but no one was quite certain what to do.

Federal officials seemed to approach the epidemic with embarrassment, declaring that the problem was a local issue; local authorities claimed they could do little without national support. Words and endless meetings became a substitute for rational action. Politicians handled the epidemic with unaccustomed wariness. Almost without exception public leaders evaded the epidemic, avoiding even the usual expressions of compassion and concern. It was as if the sexual orientation of the victims made any involvement risky, and the politicians directed their courage and energies elsewhere.

Still the young men continued to die. As of mid-April 1983, 1,339 people have been diagnosed as having AIDS. Five hundred and five cases were fatal. In New York City alone, there have been 595 cases, with 228 deaths. But even as the disaster escalated, the organized medical community was strangely absent. When a fatal infection had struck down veterans attending an American Legion convention, health professionals across the country joined in the search for a solution. When women using tampons became ill with toxic shock syndrome, medical societies and research centers immediately focused their enormous talents on that problem. But when the victims were drug addicts and poor Haitian refugees and homosexual men, their plight did not, somehow, seem as significant to those expected to speak for the health professions. No major research programs were announced, and until it became clear that the disease could spread to the general population through blood transfusions, organized medicine seemed part of the curious conspiracy of silence.

Nevertheless, when historians reflect on this epidemic, years hence, I suspect they will not stress the sordid stories of failure and neglect, but rather recount the remarkable tales of heroism that illuminate this dark, lonely period of struggle to unravel the unknown.

While government and organized medicine appeared to look for excuses for inaction, a new collective strength was building among those most at risk of contracting AIDS. Their greatest strength lay in a determination not to be destroyed, in a will that demanded public attention be paid to this epidemic, and in an unprecedented willingness to help those who needed the medical, psychological, and social assistance that society had not offered. Out of such determination was formed the Gay Men's Health Crisis, a group that has done superb work educating, advising, and sustaining frightened, vulnerable people with nowhere else to turn.

No one has captured better than Albert Camus the unique exile an epidemic imposes. In *The Plague,* he wrote:

> . . . There was always something missing in their lives. Hostile to the past, impatient of the present, and cheated of the future, we were much like those whom men's justice, or hatred, forces to live behind prison bars. . . . The plague had swallowed up everything and everyone. No longer were there individual destinies, only a collective destiny, made of plague and the emotions shared by all. Strongest of these emotions was the sense of exile and of deprivation, with all the crosscurrents of revolt and fear set up by these.

All too often the victims of AIDS have been made to feel like Camus' victims, exiled and deprived of the full measure of what modern medicine can offer. But there have also been many instances of individual courage, of simple adherence by physicians and nurses and technicians to a code as old as medicine itself. These will never be recorded or acknowledged individually. Clinical medicine is not built on heroic deeds or memorable feats but on steady, loyal service to patients. When those patients are dying in large numbers and when the mode of transmission of their disease is unknown, then the daily routine of involved health workers assumes a quiet dignity and decency that deserves special respect.

The clinician has a privileged role in an epidemic, for he shares, uniquely, the victims' sufferings, their despair, and their dwindling hopes. In this epidemic, we, as physicians, have had daily to face patients in the prime of life who are suffering from a disease we do not understand and cannot cure. We have often had to sustain them solely with the ancient commitment of our profession to remain at our posts, seeking answers and offering help until this modern plague has been conquered.

Added to the medical challenge has been a growing crisis in hospitals and social service departments faced with large numbers of AIDS patients. Because of the need for isolation precautions, every facet of their care—from nursing and nutrition to laboratory work and housekeeping—becomes extremely costly. The duration of an AIDS hospital stay is usually measured in months, and hospital bills in excess of $100,000 occur with ever-increasing frequency. Health insurance coverage for the young and poor, who constitute the majority of AIDS victims, is usually inadequate, often nonexistent. Society had not planned for this epidemic.

To address some of these problems, a group of nationally known medical specialists recently gathered in New York City for a symposium on AIDS that resulted in this book. Each participant brought a special perspective to this most complex problem. The symposium participants came to New York with the hope that their shared knowledge and experience might suggest promising avenues of investigation for researchers, lend practical aid to clinicians, and chart a course out of this crisis. The history of medicine reassures us that, with time and effort, the terrible mystery of AIDS will be unraveled and a cure found. I have no doubt that those whose words are presented here will have been major actors in bringing this life-and-death drama to an end.

When that day comes, we may look back and reflect with the same satisfaction that Camus' character, Dr. Rieux, experienced as the epidemic finally vanished from Oran:

> And it was in the midst of shouts rolling against the terrace wall in massive waves that waxed in volume and duration, while cataracts of colored fire fell thicker through the darkness, that Dr. Rieux resolved to compile this chronicle, so that he should not be one of those who hold their peace but should bear witness in favor of those plague-stricken people; so that some memorial of the injustice and outrage done them might endure; and to state quite simply what we learn in time of pestilence: that there are more things to admire in men than to despise.

Part I

Epidemiology

The solution to any mystery usually follows the accumulation of many bits of evidence and the reconstruction of the event by experts trained to create a coherent picture from apparently unrelated elements. The search by a police detective to link the method and the motive of a crime with a particular suspect has its counterpart in modern medicine in the work of the epidemiologist. He studies the patterns of illness, defines the probable path of a disease, and, thereby, helps develop programs to arrest the spread of an epidemic.

The world's leading institution in this critical science is our national Centers for Disease Control (CDC) of the U.S. Public Health Service. For the past six years, Dr. William Foege has been the Director of the CDC. His chapter on AIDS is an historic one for it is his final contribution as administrative chief of CDC. This world-renowned medical detective has elected to retire so that he can devote his full energies to the pursuit of the causes of disease. His predecessor at CDC, Dr. David Sencer, now serves as New York City's Commissioner of Health. Dr. Sencer, therefore, finds himself once again at the critical center of an epidemic, for AIDS has affected more New Yorkers than anyone else. One of the puzzling pieces in the yet unresolved enigma of AIDS is the prevalence of the syndrome in Haitian nationals and refugees. Dr. Sheldon Landesman has served as Director of the Haitian AIDS Study Group at the Downstate Medical Center in Brooklyn, New York. His chapter reflects his own experiences with Haitians in Brooklyn, and reviews the information available from Haiti and Miami.

1

The National Pattern of AIDS

William Foege, M.D.

In May 1981, CDC began investigating reports of a disease that, as of April 5, 1983, has been reported to affect more than 1,300 individuals in the United States; 489 of them have died. The patients have been found in thirty-six states, although most of them live on the East or West coast—New York, California, New Jersey, or Florida.

Although Acquired Immune Deficiency Syndrome (AIDS) has become well known through scientific publications and the mass media, its cause is not known, its exact method of transmission is not known, and the ultimate measure of its toll in deaths is not known.

Physicians are now recognizing signs and symptoms of AIDS in an increasing number of patients. In many cases, early manifestations include unexplained weight loss, night sweats, generalized lymphadenopathy, and general malaise. However, the basic disorder appears to be a defective immune system, which is no longer able to protect the body against infection and at least one type of cancer.

The first reported cases of the new syndrome were recorded in the *Morbidity and Mortality Weekly Report (MMWR)* of June 5, 1981. Five young men, all active homosexuals, had been treated in Los Angeles hospitals for a rare infection, *Pneumocystis carinii* pneumonia (PCP). Two of these five patients had died. All had evidence of other infections and a defective immune system.

The editorial note of the *MMWR* gave a hint of the puzzle that has since developed into one of the major public health and scientific challenges of this generation:

> *Pneumocystis* pneumonia in the United States is almost exclusively limited to severely immunosuppressed patients. The occurrence of pneumocystosis in 5 previously healthy individuals without a clinically apparent underlying immunodeficiency is unusual. The fact that these patients were all homosexuals suggests an association between some aspect of a homosexual lifestyle, or disease acquired through sexual contact, and *Pneumocystis* pneumonia in this population.

At about the same time, physicians diagnosed Kaposi's sarcoma, an uncommon malignancy in the United States, in 26 homosexual men— 20 in New York City and 6 in California. The 26 patients ranged in age from 26 to 51 years. Eight of the patients had died—all within 24 months after diagnosis of the unusual cancer. In June 1981, CDC began systematic surveillance for individuals with these diseases. A task force was established within CDC by July 1981 to characterize the syndrome, to determine the frequency of its occurrence in the population, to determine who was at risk of becoming ill, and why. The initial search was for laboratory-proven Kaposi's sarcoma and/or proven life-threatening opportunistic infections in previously healthy people between the ages of 15 and 60. The task force began its search by contacting physicians, other medical specialists, major hospitals, and tumor registries in New York State, California, and Georgia. Members of the task force reviewed requests made to CDC for pentamidine, a drug used to treat *Pneumocystis carinii* pneumonia and available only from CDC. Later, a surveillance system based on telephone and mail reports from individual physicians and health departments, and continuing review of requests for pentamidine, was started; this surveillance still continues.

In September 1981, a case control study was also begun. Interviews were conducted with homosexual AIDS patients and with the controls, healthy men who were homosexual and, as nearly as possible, like the patients in other ways. Fifty patients with AIDS and 120 healthy homosexual men, located through private physicians or VD clinics, were interviewed. From these interviews came some answers to the question of who was at greatest risk of developing AIDS.

Epidemiologists identified a subset of homosexual men who were more likely to have many anonymous sexual partners, to have a history of a variety of sexually transmitted diseases, and to engage in sexual practices that increased the risk of exposure to small amounts of blood and feces. The most important variable was that the AIDS patients had more male sexual partners than the controls, an average of 60 per year for patients compared with 25 per year for controls.

Meanwhile, investigators were finding AIDS in other groups of the American population. During the fall of 1981, physicians in New York treated several cases of *Pneumocystis* pneumonia and other opportunistic infections in heterosexual men and women who abused intravenous drugs. The New York and New Jersey state health departments reported a small number of prisoners with similar symptoms. About the same time, physicians in Miami reported AIDS in several Haitian patients who had recently moved to the United States. Haitians with this disease were also being seen in Brooklyn, New York.

AIDS was also diagnosed in patients with hemophilia A. In early 1982, the first report of a hemophiliac dying of PCP came from Miami. Other reports soon followed. Of these cases, the *Morbidity and Mortality Weekly Report* for July 16, 1982, said: "The clinical and immunologic features these three patients share are strikingly similar to those recently observed among certain individuals from the following groups: homosexual males, heterosexuals who abuse IV [intravenous] drugs, and Haitians who recently entered the United States. Although the cause of the severe immune dysfunction is unknown, the occurrence among the three hemophiliac cases suggests the possible transmission of an agent through blood products." In most instances, these patients have been the first AIDS cases in their cities, states, or regions. They have had no common medications, occupations, habits, or types of pets, or any uniform antecedent history of personal or family illnesses with immunological relevance.

In July 1982, representatives of CDC, the Food and Drug Administration, the National Hemophilia Foundation, and other organizations met to plan studies to evaluate the risks to hemophiliacs and to develop ways to make safer blood products for use in treating hemophilia. CDC notified directors of hemophilia centers about these cases and, with the National Hemophilia Foundation, initiated collaborative surveillance. A Public Health Service advisory committee was formed to consider the implication of these findings.

By December 1982, all three of the initial AIDS patients with hemophilia had died, and four additional heterosexual hemophilia patients had developed one or more opportunistic infections accompanied by evidence of cellular immune deficiency. Data from inquiries about the hemophilia patients' sexual activities, drug usage, travel, and residence provided no suggestion that disease could have been acquired through contact with each other, with homosexuals, with illicit drug abusers, or with Haitian immigrants. All had received Factor VIII concentrates (a blood-clotting protein), and all but one had received other blood components. (When interpreting this information, it is important to recognize that a single lot of Factor VIII concentrate may be prepared from the blood of as many as 20,000 donors.) As of April 5, 1983, CDC has received reports of AIDS in a total of 11 hemophilia patients who were not homosexual, abusers of intravenous drugs, or Haitian, and 8 of these patients have died.

The current CDC surveillance definition of AIDS requires the presence of a disease at least moderately indicative of defective cell-mediated immunity in an individual who has no known underlying cause for such a defect or any other reason for diminished resistance to that disease. Such diseases include Kaposi's sarcoma (KS) and PCP or other serious opportunistic infections. Diagnoses are considered to fit the case definition only if based on sufficiently reliable methods, generally histological or microbiological examinations. However, some patients with less well-defined manifestations of AIDS may be excluded from this surveillance definition. These manifestations may range from absence of symptoms despite laboratory evidence of immune deficiency to nonspecific symptoms (fever, weight loss, generalized or persistent lymphadenopathy) to specific diseases that are insufficiently predictive of cellular immunodeficiency to be included in incidence monitoring. Such diseases would include tuberculosis, oral candidiasis, herpes zoster, or malignant neoplasms that cause, as well as result from, immune deficiency. Conversely, some individuals who are considered AIDS patients on the basis of diseases only moderately indicative of cellular immune deficiency may not actually have an immune deficiency and may not be part of the current epidemic. In the absence of a reliable, inexpensive, widely available test for AIDS, applying the working surveillance definition appears to be the best currently available method of monitoring the incidence of AIDS.

The incidence of AIDS by date of diagnosis, assuming an almost constant population at risk of getting the disease, has roughly doubled every six months since the second half of 1979. In September 1982, more than two cases were being diagnosed every day; by March 1983, an average of four or five reports were being received by CDC each day (Figure 1). The lower number of cases recorded in the last month

FIGURE 1

ACQUIRED IMMUNE DEFICIENCY SYNDROME (AIDS)
KAPOSI'S SARCOMA (KS), PNEUMOCYSTIS PNEUMONIA (PCP),
AND OTHER OPPORTUNISTIC INFECTIONS (OI), UNITED STATES,
1979-1983, AS OF APRIL 1, 1983

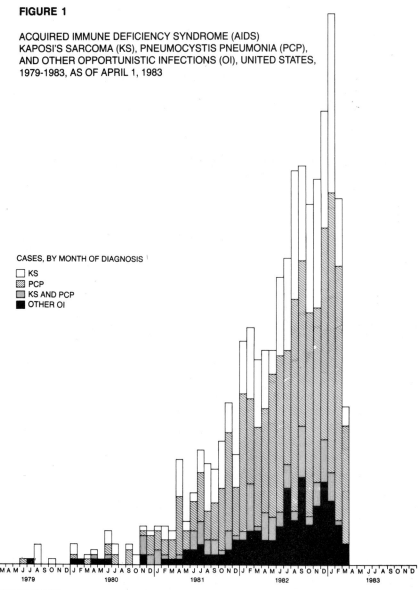

CASES, BY MONTH OF DIAGNOSIS

☐ KS
▨ PCP
▦ KS AND PCP
■ OTHER OI

1 CASE IN 1975/4 CASES 1978

shown in the figure reflects a delay between diagnosis and the receipt of all reports at CDC.

By April 5, 1983, CDC had received reports of 1,300 AIDS cases from 35 states and the District of Columbia. Almost 80 percent of reported AIDS cases in the United States are concentrated in six metropolitan areas, predominantly on the East and West coasts. These include New York City, San Francisco, Miami, Newark, and Los Angeles (Table 1). The distribution of cases is not only a reflection of population size in those areas; the number of cases per million persons in residence in New York City and San Francisco is roughly 10 times greater than that of the entire country. CDC has also received reports of 81 cases from 16 other countries.

The distribution of the 1,300 reported AIDS patients among high-risk groups is as follows: homosexual or bisexual men—72 percent; intravenous drug abusers with no history of male homosexual activity—25 percent; Haitians with a history of neither homosexuality nor intravenous drug abuse—6 percent; persons with hemophilia A who were not Haitians, homosexuals, or intravenous drug abusers—1 percent, and persons in none of the other groups—6 percent (Figure 2). The sum of these percentages slightly exceeds 100 because some of these groups are not mutually exclusive, as shown in Figure 2.

The ultimate case-fatality ratio for patients with AIDS cannot be accurately determined yet, because death from complications of this syndrome may not occur for a number of years after illness onset. Of

Table 1

Reported Cases of AIDS by Standard Metropolitan Statistical Area (SMSA) of Residence, June 1, 1981, to April 5, 1983, United States

SMSA of Residence	Cases	Percentage of Total Cases	Cases per Million Population*
New York City	603	46.4	66.1
San Francisco	164	12.6	50.5
Los Angeles	93	7.2	12.4
Miami	50	3.8	30.8
Newark	32	2.4	16.2
Elsewhere, U.S.A.	358	27.5	1.8
Total	1,300	100.0%	5.7

*Based on 1980 Census data.

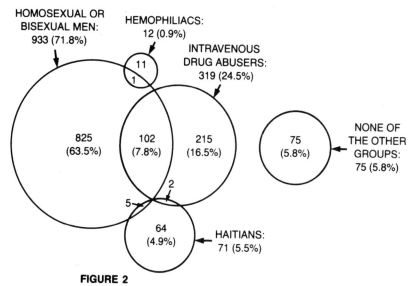

FIGURE 2

The First 1,300 Reported Cases of AIDS
in the United States, April 5, 1983:
Groups at Increased
Risk for AIDS

the 1,300 cases reported to CDC by April 5, 1983, 489 (38 percent) have been fatal. During this interval, the case-fatality ratio for patients with PCP without KS (43 percent) is twice that for patients with KS without PCP (21 percent), while the risk of death for patients with both PCP and KS (50 percent) is even higher (Table 2). The eventual AIDS case-fatality ratio several years after diagnosis may be far greater. Of the 51 patients diagnosed in 1979–80, 44 (86 percent) are now dead (Table 3).

The occurrence of generalized lymphadenopathy in patients with manifestations of systemic illness, such as weight loss and malaise, but without KS, PCP, or other opportunistic infections, may represent a prodromal phase of AIDS. Many physicians have reported seeing an increase in the number of homosexual men with chronic, unexplained, diffuse lymphadenopathy. Some, but not all, of these men have cellular immune deficiency. A small proportion of these patients have later developed KS or opportunistic infections.

Additionally, investigators from New York City have described the occurrence of abnormalities of cellular immune function, usually mild,

Table 2

Reported AIDS Cases and Case-Fatality Ratios, by Disease Category, for Cases Reported June 1, 1981, to April 5, 1983, United States

Disease Category	Cases		Deaths		Case-Fatality Ratio
	No.	% of Total	No.	% of Total	
KS without PCP	357	(27.5)	75	(15.3)	21%
PCP without KS	656	(50.4)	282	(57.7)	43%
Both KS and PCP	104	(8.0)	52	(10.6)	50%
Other opportunistic infections	183	(14.1)	80	(16.4)	44%
Total	1,300	(100.0)	489	(100.0)	38%

Table 3

Reported Cases of AIDS and Case-Fatality Ratios by Half-Year of Diagnosis, 1979 to 1983, United States, as of April 5, 1983

		Number of Cases	Number of Deaths	Case-Fatality Ratio
1979	Jan.–June	1	1	100%
	July–Dec.	7	5	71%
1980	Jan.–June	18	14	78%
	July–Dec.	25	24	96%
1981	Jan.–June	70	54	77%
	July–Dec.	148	106	72%
1982	Jan.–June	292	127	43%
	July–Dec.	488	121	25%
1983	Jan.–Apr. 5	240	33	14%

in apparently healthy homosexual men. The natural history of this "subclinical immunosuppression" is unknown.

It is possible that AIDS may cause other disease manifestations in homosexual men. For example, some physicians have reported the occurrence of autoimmune thrombocytopenic purpura in homosexual men with cellular immunodeficiency. An apparent excess of several other highly unusual malignancies, such as diffuse undifferentiated non-Hodgkin's lymphoma and lymphoma of the brain, has been reported in young homosexual men.

Based on current information, AIDS appears to be caused by an infectious agent. The transmission of AIDS appears most commonly to require intimate, direct contact involving mucosal surfaces, such as sexual contact between homosexual males. Parenteral spread, such as occurs with intravenous drug abusers and possibly hemophilia patients using Factor VIII concentrate, would also seem a probable route of transmission. Airborne spread and interpersonal spread through casual contact do not seem likely. These patterns resemble the distribution of disease and modes of spread of hepatitis B virus (HBV), and hepatitis B virus infections occur very frequently in AIDS cases.

The occurrence of disease among intravenous drug users who share potentially contaminated needles and hemophiliacs who receive blood products suggests a viremic state. Whether the duration of this putative viremia is short or long remains to be seen, but it seems unlikely that a short infection would produce such a persistent and progressive T cell abnormality.

Evidence that AIDS may be caused by an infectious agent, including the similarity of its epidemiological course to that of hepatitis B, has made it necessary to develop recommendations or precautions for clinical and laboratory staff members who might come in contact with such an agent. These precautions are similar to the ones medical and hospital personnel are asked to observe when working with hepatitis B patients.

If the theory is correct that AIDS is caused by a virus, health workers having parenteral exposure to blood from AIDS patients need to be watched for any signs and symptoms of the disease. The rate of occurrence of disease in affected groups will be a function of the transmissibility of the agent within each group, the presence of preexisting immunity, if any, and the incubation period of the disease. That period now appears to be twelve months or more.

Another observation that raised concern over the possible role of blood in the transmission of AIDS was the report of severe immune deficiency and opportunistic infection appearing in an infant several months after transfusion of platelets derived from the blood of a man who, although apparently well, subsequently developed AIDS. Several other similar observations have raised the possibility that blood may be a vehicle for transmitting AIDS.

On the basis of evidence that AIDS was apparently occurring for the first time in patients with hemophilia, and with preliminary evidence that blood transfusions might be implicated in the transmission of AIDS, the health community developed recommendations aimed at preventing transmission of AIDS through the use of blood products. The National Gay Task Force, the National Hemophilia Foundation, the American Red Cross, the American Association of Blood Banks, the Council of Community Blood Centers, the American Association of Physicians for Human Rights, and others issued statements about the prevention and control of AIDS.

On March 4, 1983, the Public Health Service recommended the following actions to reduce the risk of contracting AIDS:

1. Sexual contact should be avoided with persons known or suspected to have AIDS. Members of high-risk groups should be aware that multiple sexual partners increase the probability of developing AIDS.

2. As a temporary measure, members of groups at increased risk for AIDS should refrain from donating plasma and/or blood. This recommendation includes all individuals belonging to such groups, even though many individuals are at little risk of AIDS. Centers collecting plasma and/or blood should inform potential donors of this recommendation. The Food and Drug Administration is preparing new recommendations for manufacturers of plasma derivatives and for establishments collecting plasma or blood. This is an interim measure to protect recipients of blood products and blood until specific laboratory tests are available.

3. Studies should be conducted to evaluate screening procedures for their effectiveness in identifying and excluding plasma and blood with a high probability of transmitting AIDS. The procedures should include specific laboratory tests as well as careful histories and physical examinations.

4. Physicians should adhere strictly to medical indications for transfusions, and autologous blood transfusions are encouraged.

5. Work should continue toward development of safer blood products for use by hemophilia patients.

Laboratory work on AIDS has brought to light as many puzzling questions as has the epidemiology of the disease. The first and most apparent link between the varied groups of AIDS patients was the immune defect observed. Patients with AIDS have normal or elevated concentrations of serum antibodies and of the cells that produce antibody. Certain types of white blood cells, called helper T cells (T_H), are abnormally low in number. By contrast, suppressor T cells (T_S) are present in normal or increased numbers, resulting in a lower than normal ratio of T_H to T_S cells.

Herpesviruses, most notably Epstein-Barr virus and cytomegalovirus (CMV), can infect circulating and noncirculating lymphocytes and cause persistent infections. Thus, herpesviruses could fulfill some of the criteria required of an agent causing AIDS. CMV has been suggested as a cause of AIDS by several investigators, although in several patients there is inconclusive evidence of previous CMV infection, based on laboratory data now available. Human T cell leukemia virus (HTLV) is also transmitted person-to-person, is found to infect individuals in clusters, and is associated with the development of cancer after a long period of time. This virus infects T helper cells and apparently alters their function to that of a suppressor cell. The adult T cell leukemia/lymphoma, which occurs at increased rates in areas where HTLV is endemic, has been described by the Japanese as a new disease. Although HTLV is not widely prevalent in the United States, scientists are examining what role, if any, this or similar agents might have in causing AIDS or illness among patients with AIDS.

Assuming that the infectious agent hypothesis is correct, what will the future hold? A continued increase of cases may be expected among homosexual men. If the HBV model is a valid one, the sexual partners of affected heterosexual men and women may become infected. If blood from infected individuals can transmit disease, recipients of other blood products may contract AIDS.

In summary, during the past two years, an epidemic of devastating illnesses has been taking place in the United States. These diseases include fatal opportunistic infections, Kaposi's sarcoma, and perhaps other cancers and illnesses. These diseases have afflicted young homosexual men predominantly. The reported incidence of AIDS has continued to rise steadily, and only 19 percent of the known patients have survived two years or longer after diagnosis.

The tragedy of the AIDS epidemic is intensified by the youth of the victims, the lack of proven treatments, and the prolonged, costly, debilitating, and often fatal illnesses that occur. The median age of the patients has been 34 years; 92 percent are below the age of 50. Many productive years have been prematurely lost to this epidemic. Many patients have survived one illness only to suffer a fatal recurrence of infection or to develop a fatal cancer.

This epidemic offers a unique scientific challenge to better understand the human immune system and its role in controlling cancer and infection, but more importantly it provides a mandate to learn the causes of AIDS, so that the suffering and deaths caused by these illnesses can be prevented.

2

Tracking a Local Outbreak

David J. Sencer, M.D.

New York City has the unhappy distinction of having more cases of AIDS diagnosed and reported in residents than any other city in the United States. About one-half of all cases in the United States are consistently reported from New York City. At this time (April 10, 1983) there are over 600 cases of AIDS confirmed in New York City's five boroughs. There are those who argue that the number of reported cases is high here in part because New York physicians are more apt than others to recognize the syndrome. That view is countered somewhat by our experience. Within recent weeks a concentrated effort of active surveillance has actually increased the number of previously unreported cases.

The epidemic shows no evidence of waning. The epidemic curve pictured in Figure 1 should not be misread to indicate a downward trend in cases. This histogram notes the number of cases by date of onset of symptoms. One must read it bearing in mind that there is a temporal lag between onset of symptoms and the seeking of medical advice, between the confirmation of diagnosis and reporting. The true picture is one of a constantly increasing incidence, as seen in Figure 2, where the cases have been accumulated by quarter of calendar years. Table 1 shows the trends in cases reported and diagnosed by month for the past nine months.

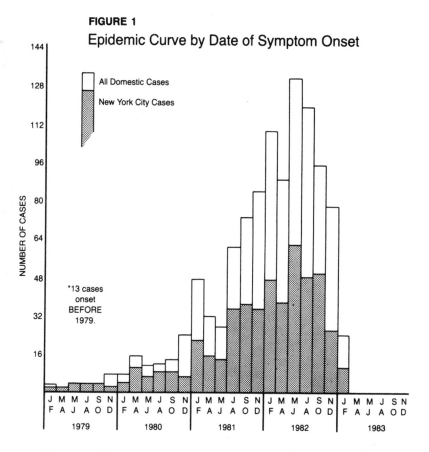

FIGURE 1

Epidemic Curve by Date of Symptom Onset

Our surveillance measures take into account the usual factors, such as place of residence. There is a predominance of cases in residents of Manhattan (Figure 3). This is not surprising when one considers that three-quarters of the cases reported nationwide to date have been in male homosexuals and that there are large concentrations of male homosexuals in the borough of Manhattan.

There are variations in reported cases by ethnic group (Table 2). Of particular significance is the number of patients of Haitian origin. Although no accurate census of Haitians in New York City is available, the number of cases appears to be in excess of that expected.

The age distribution of the New York City cases is no different from that of the rest of the country, with a median age of 34 years.

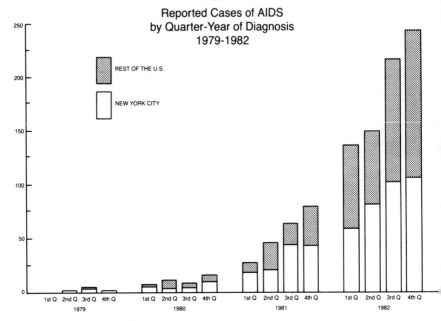

FIGURE 2

Reported Cases of AIDS
by Quarter-Year of Diagnosis
1979-1982

Table 1

New York City Surveillance
Trends: AIDS Cases by Month

Month	Number Diagnosed	Number Reported
1982		
July	29	35
August	36	39
September	38	34
October	44	29
November	35	46
December	31	37
1983		
January	48	50
February	22	58
March	29	61

FIGURE 3

Breakdown by Residence of Cases on NYC Computer

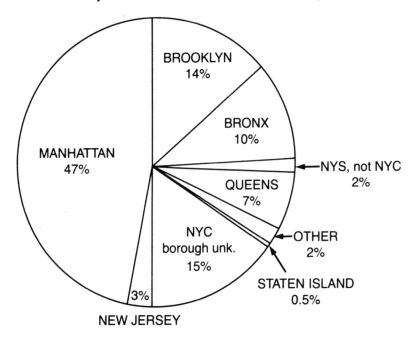

Table 2

AIDS Cases by Race, N.Y.C. (Male and Female), February 16, 1983

Race	% of Total Cases
White	52%
Black	25%
Hispanic	19%
Haitian	3%
Other	1%
Unknown	1%

These are the typical demographic factors measured by surveillance, but with the advent of this disease we have had to take into account "sociodemographic" risk factors not usually applied in a surveillance situation. In New York City 69 percent of reported cases are in homosexual and bisexual males and 22 percent in drug abusers (Table 3). The drug abusers have all been hard-core heroin users, not occasional social users of drugs. Fifteen percent of the drug users who contracted AIDS are females; that number accounts for 62 percent of all female AIDS cases reported in New York City. We have had no reported cases among hemophiliacs at this time; this is not surprising when analyzed statistically.

The New York City distribution of cases by primary diagnosis and sex, shown in Table 4, is in keeping with that which is seen in other parts of the country.

It was previously thought that 28 people in New York City who were in none of the at-risk categories had contracted AIDS. These cases have now been analyzed and narrowed down to a relatively few who appear to be neither within the at-risk groups nor to have had contact with susceptible individuals (Table 5).

The lethal nature of this disease can be realized by the mortality trend that we have observed in New York City. By the end of the third year of observation and treatment of cases in New York City, 60 percent of those who have been diagnosed were dead; by the end of

Table 3

New York City Surveillance
Cases by Risk Group, Males and Females, April 13, 1983

Risk Group	Number	% of Total Cases
Homosexual or bisexual	446	69%
IV drug user (no history of homosexuality)	139	22%
Haitian (no history of homosexuality or IV drug use)	22	4%
Hemophiliac	0	0
Other	35	5%
Total	642*	100%

*Five females are not included here because of a coding error in collecting data.

Table 4

New York City Surveillance—Reported Cases
March 9–April 9, 1983

Males	New Cases	Total Cases	% Total Male Cases
Kaposi's sarcoma (KS)	11	222	38%
Pneumocystis carinii pneumonia (PCP) without KS	25	276	46%
Other OI (without KS or PCP)	17	99	16%
Total males	53	597	100%

Females	New Cases	Total Cases	% Total Female Cases
KS	1	4	8%
PCP	4	28	56%
OI	4	18	36%
Total females	9	50	
Total cases	64	647	100%

CDC National Surveillance (April 13, 1983):
Total domestic cases: 1339
Total foreign cases: 84

Table 5

New York City Surveillance
AIDS Cases Without Apparent "Risk Factors"

I. Cases deceased prior to interview—risk factor status unknown.	13
II. Probable "background" KS cases.	2
III. Intimate contact with an "at-risk" group.	7
IV. Possible transfusion-associated cases.	2
V. Interviewed—without risk factors.	4
Total	28

1981, 56 percent; and by the end of 1982, 43 percent (Table 6). This disease has one of the highest case-fatality rates of any infectious disease of man that has been described.

The purpose of all our surveillance activities at the Health Department is not simply the compilation of statistics. We hope through this descriptive epidemiology to find a way of preventing the spread of AIDS. It was by such a process that John Snow in 1853 was able to end a cholera epidemic then sweeping through parts of London. He found that all the victims drank water from one particular pump on Broad Street. He removed the handle of the Broad Street pump and put an end to the epidemic, thirty years before the causative agent of cholera was isolated by Robert Koch.

Apart from the traditional epidemiologic challenges, this epidemic has brought with it some unique problems and has engendered some unique responses from government officials and others. These, I think, are worthy of note.

Each of the at-risk groups identified in New York City—homosexually active males, intravenous drug abusers, and Haitians—is outside the mainstream of society either racially or through social behavior. There is no need to rehearse here the evidences of discrimination against these groups. Their association with this disease has, in some instances, heightened the discrimination that, in more or less subtle ways, they experience.

Table 6

Trends:
AIDS Cases by Half-Year of Diagnosis, N.Y.C.

	Number Diagnosed	Percent Dead
1st half 1978	4	50%
2nd half 1978	1	0
1st half 1979	1	100%
2nd half 1979	5	80%
1st half 1980	10	40%
2nd half 1980	14	71%
1st half 1981	39	67%
2nd half 1981	86	50%
1st half 1982	135	27%
2nd half 1982	191	30%

Questions arise about employing gays or Haitians. A Haitian schoolteacher tells me that children of Haitian origin are being taunted in the schools because of the connection in the scientific literature and the public media between Haitians and AIDS. I do not need to dwell upon the fact that intravenous drug abusers are not integrated into our society—in fact, they are often referred to as a "subculture."

We should remember, too, that each of the at-risk groups may be suspicious of outsiders, including public health and health care workers. In addition, most public health workers—being non-gay, non-Haitian, and non–drug abusers—may be ignorant of the life-styles and practices of these groups and have difficulty communicating effectively with those suffering from or at risk of AIDS. We are therefore faced with epidemiologic problems that transcend merely the usual investigation of an outbreak of a new disease. We are faced with not only defining the disease and searching for the agent, but with eliminating the barriers of discrimination, ignorance, and mistrust that may separate victims from investigators. I had a professor who said that the problem most public health workers had in communicating was that they were from middle- or upper-class income and educational environments while their clientele were of a lower socioeconomic group. That analysis, with some variations, applies well here.

Despite these problems, New York City is uniquely equipped to address this major geographical focus of AIDS. We have a highly effective health research and health care system that rapidly recognized the severity and magnitude of the problem. In an effort to improve communications among the multiple institutions working in the field, the Health Department began, a little over a year ago, offering itself as a convening ground where investigators could share their findings and speed the interchange of scientific information. Monthly meetings were initiated. After the first, rather stilted meeting, where everyone was keeping their own findings quite close to their vests, there has been a tremendous outpouring of information in these meetings. To me they have been unique in that the research community has recognized that they are interdependent upon each other rather than independent and that by sharing information, answers will be more rapidly achieved.

Another phenomenon has taken place in New York City that I think is as unique as the sharing of research information. This is the development within the gay community of a Scientific Advisory Committee that offers itself to review research proposals in a peer review capacity and also as a means of attempting to ensure that the rights of the community are protected. The concept of informed consent by the individual is by now a well-accepted doctrine, and in most medical centers there are institutional review boards that control all aspects of human research projects. However, involvement of an affected community in the collection and interpretation of data relevant to their own health is, to me, an important new venture in epidemiology. This approach enhances the credibility of investigators and minimizes the risk of misunderstanding the population being investigated. At the New York City Health Department we have established as policy that we will undertake no investigations without the participation of the above-mentioned Scientific Advisory Committee with the Department of Health's institutional review board.

We have also established a group composed of representatives from city agencies involved in providing services to present or potential patients with AIDS and of representatives from risk groups. This group meets monthly and has served to identify problems and solve some. The first several meetings limited themselves to meeting with representatives from the gay community, but at our next meeting we hope to have individuals who can speak to the concerns of the other population groups who are principally at risk, namely the Haitian community and the drug abuse population. As an epidemiologist, I feel we need this type of crosscommunication in order that we can be more precise in our definition of the population at risk. Some case-control studies have shown that not all male homosexuals are at equal risk but that there may be behavioral, environmental, or host factors that predispose certain individuals to be at higher risk. Similar studies need to be undertaken in the other major risk groups for two reasons: the epidemiological purpose of better understanding the disease process, and the social purpose of reducing some of the discriminatory practices against these population groups as a result of their association with AIDS.

To assist the Health Department in better understanding and communicating with the major population group at risk in New York City, we have established an Office of Gay and Lesbian Health Concerns. While this office is principally concerned today with the problems of AIDS, the longer-term goals are to better integrate into the health care system those who are now discriminated against. This office will be concerned, among other things, with developing educational programs for ensuring that appropriate services are available both in the public and voluntary sectors. It will act as a focal point for concerns that are raised from the gay and lesbian communities. It is our aim not to duplicate or segmentize services but to ensure that the services are open to all regardless of race, creed, color, country of origin, or sexual orientation.

The history of public health is replete with incidents of discriminatory barriers causing lack of services, both preventive and curative, and thereby the continuation of disease transmission. In any epidemic, such actions are wrong. Faced with a disease of the magnitude and severity of AIDS, we cannot allow person-constructed barriers to interfere with the rapid achievement of our aim: to find and remove the handle from the Broad Street pump of this disease.

3

The Haitian Connection

Sheldon H. Landesman, M.D.

Introduction

To the American imagination, Haiti is an exotic land full of contrast and contradiction where wealth lives adjacent to abject poverty, voodoo flourishes amid Catholicism, and a sophisticated French-educated elite govern an illiterate peasantry. It is understandable, therefore, that when AIDS started to claim Haitians as victims, the juxtaposition of a mystifying disease with an exotic culture created a great deal of media attention and speculation. The scientific facts relevant to AIDS in Haitians have been lost amid the speculative ideas that have circulated. My purpose here, then, is to review briefly a few pertinent facts about Haitian culture and society and to state clearly what is known and what is not known about AIDS in Haitians, what questions need to be asked by investigators here and in Haiti.

Haitian Culture

Haitian society is a two-tiered structure. The top tier, composed of the bureaucrats, technocrats, and professionals who run the country, is well educated, Catholic, and French-speaking. Their orientation is continental, specifically French. Many of them receive their education in France. The lower tier comprises 90 percent of the population and is made up of the politically powerless farmers who speak Creole, practice voodoo, and barely survive in an economy based on a subsistence agriculture. The Haitian farmer is the poorest in Latin America and one of the poorest in the world, with an average income of less than $100 per year. It is important to note that the cultural characteristics of the two tiers are not absolutely rigid. Many educated Haitians speak Creole in addition to French, and many farmers practice Catholicism as well as voodoo, a religious system that encompasses elements of Catholic and West African rituals. In the United States, the cultural, religious, and economic separation of the two tiers persists, although the more open nature of American society has allowed for some upward mobility.

The exact number of Haitians in this country is unknown and unknowable. (Current estimates are in the range of 400,000 to 500,000.) Except for a small group of Haitians who came to the United States in the 1920s, no immigration occurred until after 1957, when Dr. Francois "Papa Doc" Duvalier became president of Haiti. At that time many of his political opponents fled to the United States with the hope of eventually going back to Haiti to oust Dr. Duvalier from power by military means. But Duvalier retained power until his death, when his son assumed the leadership. The early political refugees, many of whom were from upper-class Haitian families, became permanent residents of this country.

More recently large numbers of poor Haitians, many without legal documents, have immigrated into the United States. These persons were fleeing their country more for economic than for political reasons. In contrast to the earlier immigrants, the more recent arrivals came from the impoverished rural sections of Haiti. The health status of the new immigrants mirrored their poor economic condition: tuberculosis, parasitic infestation, salmonellosis, malaria, and malnutrition were common. The total number of recent arrivals is estimated to be at least 100,000.

Large Haitian communities exist in Miami, New York City, Newark, and Montreal. Smaller communities are scattered throughout the United States. New York City contains the largest Haitian community in the country (approximately 300,000), followed by Miami (60,000 to 70,000). The Haitian community in New York City has been in this country longer, is better educated, and more representative of upper-class Haitian society than are the communities in Miami or Newark.

The Haitian community in this country is relatively closed to outsiders; Haitians usually associate only with fellow Haitians outside of their jobs. The cultural cohesiveness of the community is maintained and heightened by Haitian newspapers, radio stations, churches, and self-help organizations.

AIDS Among Haitian Immigrants to the U.S.

In June of 1981, what we now call AIDS was diagnosed nearly simultaneously in New York City, Los Angeles, and San Francisco; initially the disease was reported to occur exclusively in male homosexuals residing in these cities. Soon it became apparent that the disease also occurred in intravenous drug users, hemophiliacs, and Haitians. The Haitian cases were reported from Miami and New York City, the two cities with the largest Haitian communities in the country. The cases in Miami came from Jackson Memorial, a hospital that serves the indigent of the Miami area. In New York City large numbers of Haitians live in the Brooklyn-Queens area. Many lack health insurance and seek medical care at Kings County Hospital, the largest municipal hospital in Brooklyn and traditionally the source of health care for the poor of that borough, and the hospital there has treated the greatest number of Haitian AIDS victims. Although the bulk of the cases were seen in New York City and Miami, cases were also seen wherever there were Haitain communities, e.g., Montreal and Newark. The total number of cases among Haitian immigrants in the United States presently stands at 70. At least 20 additional cases of the putative AIDS prodrome—fever, weight loss, diarrhea, or lymphadenopathy—are under investigation.

Our experience at Kings County Hospital with Haitians is part of the grim but not atypical AIDS scenario. Twenty-one of 26 patients are dead. The proximate cause of death was *Pneumocystis carinii* pneumonia—10 cases; CNS (central nervous system) toxoplasmosis—8 cases; disseminated cryptococcal infection—3 cases. Concurrent infections included tuberculosis—6 cases; oral or esophageal candidiasis—7 cases; salmonellosis—one case. Two persons also had Kaposi's sarcoma.

AIDS in Haiti

Data on the occurrence of AIDS in Haiti is presently sparse and difficult to obtain. There are obvious logistic difficulties in collecting and processing specimens. The only published data is an abstract by

Liautaud wherein he described several cases of Kaposi's sarcoma in young, previously healthy, heterosexual Haitian males. Kaposi's sarcoma, while relatively common in equatorial West Africa, was, prior to this report, considered exceedingly rare in Haiti. Autopsy studies done in Port-au-Prince by the Centers for Disease Control and investigators from the University of Miami have documented several cases of opportunistic infection, principally central nervous system toxoplasmosis and *Pneumocystis carinii* pneumonia, in otherwise healthy Haitians. These cases have all occurred since 1979. There are reports from Haitian physicians in Port-au-Prince stating that there are large numbers of AIDS cases in that city. In these as yet unpublished reports, opportunistic infections rather than Kaposi's sarcoma were the most common manifestation of the disease.

At the present time, our knowledge about the incidence and prevalence of AIDS in Haiti is admittedly incomplete and perhaps even inaccurate. Cooperative and collaborative efforts between physicians and the government in Haiti and their counterparts here in the United States would be both useful and important in attempting to accurately ascertain the extent of the problem in Haiti. Based upon available information, it appears that AIDS does occur in Haiti—manifested by both Kaposi's sarcoma and opportunistic infections—and that the disease was not present in that country prior to 1979.

Clinical and Immunological Characteristics

Clinically, AIDS among Haitians differs from the disease in other high-risk groups in the following areas:

1. Tuberculosis is often the harbinger of the full-blown syndrome. We have had experience with several Haitian patients who first came to our attention because they had pulmonary tuberculosis, were appropriately diagnosed and treated, but often failed to respond to therapy. Several months after the initiation of therapy they went on to develop opportunistic infections characteristic of AIDS. It is our as yet unproven assumption that the development of tuberculosis in these patients was the first manifestation of waning immunity in a population where tuberculosis is endemic.

2. Kaposi's sarcoma as a manifestation of AIDS in Haitians is rare in this country. In Haiti most of the initial cases of AIDS were reported as cases of Kaposi's sarcoma. Whether this is an artifact

of reporting or represents a true difference in the manifestations of AIDS among Haitians here and in Haiti remains to be seen. When Kaposi's sarcoma occurs in Haitians, its clinical manifestation and clinical course appear to be no different from Kaposi's sarcoma in homosexuals. Studies on HLA typing to determine genetic susceptibility of Haitian persons to Kaposi's sarcoma have not yet been reported.

3. Central nervous system toxoplasmosis is more common as an opportunistic infection in Haitians with AIDS than it is in other persons with AIDS. Presumably this represents a reactivation of toxoplasmosis in a population where the disease is assumed to be endemic. To prove the above assumption, a serological survey of toxoplasmosis antibody titers in Haitians will have to be done. Such a study is presently underway.

4. Salmonellosis is seen with increased frequency in Haitians with AIDS compared to other AIDS patients. As is the case with toxoplasmosis and tuberculosis, this probably represents reactivation of endogenous infection in a host with waning immunity.

The immunological parameters in Haitians with AIDS, like the clinical characteristics of the disease, are very similar to those seen in homosexuals, intravenous drug users, and hemophiliacs. Skin test anergy, lymphopenia, reversed helper/suppressor cell ratio, decreased response to mitogens, and depressed interferon production are immunological parameters characteristic of all patients with AIDS. Taken together, these deficiencies indicate an immune system that is incapable of response to challenge.

Epidemiology

The unique aspect of AIDS in the Haitian population does not relate to the clinical manifestations or the immunological abnormalities present in these patients. Rather, it is the epidemiology of the disease in this clearly defined ethnic group that is of unusual interest. The total number of reported cases among Haitians is 70; this number is definitely an underestimate. The mean age of the patients is 30; this is 3 to 6 years younger than the mean age of homosexual and intravenous drug users with AIDS. Mean time of residence in the United States is 2.7 years, with a range from "just off the boat" to 11 years. The disease appears to be more common in the recent Haitian immigrants than in Haitians who have been in the United States for 10 years. Several of these latter cases deny recent travel to Haiti or sexual contact with recent immigrants. The fact that the recent immigrants are more likely to acquire AIDS is in accord with the epidemiological data that suggests the absence of AIDS in Haiti prior to 1979. It is obvious that intense epidemiological field work is needed in Haiti.

Approximately 80 percent of the cases are seen in presumably heterosexual male Haitians, most of them recent arrivals in this country. A breakdown of the sex of the recent immigrants shows that about 70 percent of them are male.

Essential questions to ask about the Haitians are, how did the disease first gain entry to their community, and how is it spread within the community? The answers to these questions may well be central to understanding the entire epidemiology of AIDS, perhaps even the origin of the disease. For gay males, intravenous drug users, and hemophiliacs, epidemiological evidence strongly suggests that sexual contact and blood are mechanisms by which the disease spreads. *These two mechanisms, homosexual contact, or blood, do not at present account for the introduction and spread of disease within the Haitian community*. Limited epidemiological investigation of the Haitian AIDS cases in this country indicates that homosexual practices are not the means by which the disease has been spread. Except for three cases of AIDS in admittedly homosexual Haitians, none of the other cases reported in this country have admitted to homosexual activity despite intensive questioning in both French and Creole by both American physicians and by Haitians. Although the evidence clearly suggests that homosexuality is not the mechanism of disease transmission among Haitians, this conclusion must be regarded as preliminary. Cultural and societal factors and the language barrier are real obstacles that have inhibited the collection of accurate and interpretable epidemiological facts from the Haitians. There are yet unconfirmed reports that suggest that homosexuality may be a factor in the spread of the disease within the Haitian community, but until these reports are substantiated, they must be regarded as suspect.

The second common mode of spread, through blood or blood products, does not account for the spread of the disease in the Haitian community. As far as we can tell, all of the patients seen so far were not drug addicts and, except for perhaps one, had not received blood transfusions. Questions have been raised, mostly in the popular media, that perhaps the disease is transmitted among Haitians through some spiritual or voodoo ritual. There is no evidence at present to support this contention. Among the patients we questioned and among the reports that have been received by the government, such rituals, at least at the present time, were not a factor related to the spread of the disease. What is needed is a case-control study to ascertain if any particular aspect of Haitian social behavior is associated with an increased risk of acquiring AIDS.

Severe malnutrition is a well-known cause of T cell deficiency and is associated with the development of *Pneumocystis carinii* pneumonia. Malnutrition has been postulated as a causative factor leading to AIDS in Haitians. Although malnutrition was not uncommon in recent Haitian immigrants, there is no evidence that it plays a role in the full expression of the AIDS syndrome. Some Haitians with AIDS were malnourished, but most of the protein-calorie deficiency was a consequence rather than a cause of the disease.

If homosexual contact, blood transfer, and malnutrition do not account for the presence and transmission of AIDS in Haitians, other mechanisms of transmission must be pursued. Haiti is a tropical island and it is not unreasonable to assume that transmission of the alleged "AIDS agent" is different there than in a temperate country like the United States.

Data obtained from Haitian immigrants with AIDS do not reveal any focality of disease in Haiti, i.e., the Haitian immigrants with AIDS come from geographically separate areas of Haiti. The disease is more common, however, in the urban centers of the country. If the disease is truly widespread throughout Haiti, then the possibility that an insect might be involved in the transmission is increased. It is possible that most Haitians with the disease acquired it in Haiti; after moving to this country, the disease continued to spread through normal heterosexual contact. When and if investigations are carried out in Haiti, studies on disease transmission by animal and insect vectors should be performed.

Recent reports document the occurrence of AIDS cases in equatorial Africa, particularly Zaire. It would be interesting to know about recent migration from Zaire and adjoining countries into Haiti. One can speculate that the "AIDS agent" is a virus that arose in Africa and was carried to Haiti by travelers or immigrants.

We are left then with an epidemiological void in trying to explain how the disease is spread within the Haitian population. Neither homosexual practices nor blood appear to acount for the disease within this population group. Attempts to accumulate the data that can explain the disease in this population are hampered by cultural and language barriers. Further difficulties may be encountered when trying to cross governmental and bureaucratic barriers; cooperation between Haiti and the United States, both at the higher levels of government and by medical researchers, is essential if useful information is to be discovered.

Social and Economic Impact of AIDS

A word about the impact of this disease on the Haitian community itself. Prior to the development of AIDS, the community was already upset with publications that documented a high incidence of tuberculosis and positive syphilis serology among Haitians. As a group Haitians were not happy with these publications, but their practical effect on them was limited. This has not been the case with AIDS. Recent publications documenting AIDS in Haitians, accompanied by media publicity, has had a dramatic and negative impact on the Haitian community. Haitians feel that the effect of these articles and the attendant publicity was to further brand the Haitian as a carrier of disease who ought to be avoided. This feeling was exacerbated greatly after the U.S. Public Health Service recommended that all persons at high risk for AIDS, including persons of Haitian origin, be discouraged from donating blood.

The practical impact of the scientific and media coverage of AIDS in Haitians is felt in two areas. First, members of the Haitian community themselves have become very frightened that they are at risk of acquiring the disease. Second, some Haitians have had their livelihoods threatened by the AIDS problem in their community. On several occasions we have received phone calls from prospective employers of Haitians asking if it was safe to employ them. We have advised that if the potential employee is otherwise healthy, and if his contact is not of the type where there would be sexual activity or passage of blood, then it was as safe to employ a Haitian as it was to employ anyone else in this country. Despite these reassurances, which we have put in writing to employers, we have heard of instances of Haitians losing their jobs simply because they were Haitian. This type of economic consequence is obviously not confined to Haitians alone. The same can be said for other groups afflicted, in particular homosexuals. However, homosexuals, if they so choose, can hide their sexual orientation and thus, under some circumstances, limit the economic impact associated with the occurrence of AIDS in their community. Haitians cannot hide their national origin, and thus they become the most visible targets of fear and discrimination.

It is incumbent upon physicians dealing with this disease, and upon members of the media who report on it, to act and speak with the utmost discretion and care. Because this disease is so deadly in those who have it, and so frightening to everyone, especially to those in the at-risk groups, media reports and interpretations of scientific data must be very careful and precise. If they are not, and if sensationalist aspects of this disease are played up, the result would be a general populace that is more frightened than it need be, and specific population groups discriminated against when they need not be. A cautious, responsible attitude is needed by all.

The Future

A recurrent theme of this conference is the question "Where do we go from here?" To pen what is known about AIDS is necessary but insufficient; to indicate a course to follow to solve the riddle of AIDS is the truly important task. For the "Haitian Connection," future research is more important than present knowledge. An understanding of the epidemiology of AIDS in Haitians will go far toward solving the enigma of this disease. It is useful, then, in closing this paper to summarize the known facts, emphasize our areas of ignorance, and point to a direction where the expenditure of resources, human and monetary, would reap benefits.

I. What we know
   a. AIDS does occur in Haitians, both in this country and in Haiti.
   b. The presumed modes of transmission, blood and homosexual contact, do not at present account for the introduction of AIDS into the Haitian community or its spread within the community.
   c. The clinical and immunological features of the disease are similar to those seen in homosexuals, intravenous drug users, and hemophiliacs.
   d. The disease is distinctly more common in Haitians who emigrated to this country within the last five years.
II. What we need to know
   a. How the disease entered Haiti and how it is transmitted among Haitians.
   b. What specific risk factors are associated with spread of the disease among Haitians.

III. What we have to do
   a. A case-control study.
   b. Epidemiological studies in Haiti to determine the magnitude of the problem in that country.
   c. A study in Haiti of animal and arthropod vectors.

Conclusion

A final word. The development of AIDS among non-addict, heterosexual Haitians suggests that immunity from AIDS is not conferred or guaranteed by virtue of a traditional life-style. The occurrence of AIDS in Haitians should dispel complacency that this is "just a gay disease" without serious public health ramifications for everyone. The general populace must therefore do more than just take note of the epidemic as reported in the press. They must become advocates, along with the victims, for a more aggressive governmental policy aimed at discovering the cause and a cure for the disease.

Part II

Immunology

The human immune system is an exquisitely complex mechanism that protects the body against disease. When it is functioning as it should, our immune system will identify, attack, and destroy foreign pathogenic substances. When it fails—as it does with AIDS—the body is left defenseless against an awesome array of morbid agents. Most of what we now know about this system is based on discoveries of the past quarter-century by researchers on the very frontiers of modern medicine.

Throughout a distinguished career, Dr. Robert Good has been one of the pioneers on this ever-expanding front. He is currently Head of Cancer Research and Clinical Immunology at the Oklahoma Medical Research Foundation and was formerly president and scientific director at Memorial Sloan-Kettering Cancer Center in New York. His chapter summarizes some of the most recent developments in the study of the immune system, an understanding of which is vital to the treatment of AIDS victims.

4

Immunologic Aberrations: The AIDS Defect

Robert A. Good, Ph.D., M.D.

AIDS, which appeared in epidemic form initially among homosexual males only about four years ago, is one of the most lethal of all the immunodeficiency diseases. Indeed, its lethality is rivaled only by genetically determined forms of severe combined immunodeficiency disease (SCID). Untreated SCID cases are almost always fatal before the end of the first year, and even well-treated patients whose immunodeficiency is not corrected by cellular engineering through bone marrow or fetal liver transplantation often die before the end of the second year. Because of their inordinate susceptibility to infection, one-half of patients with AIDS die before the end of the first year of their relentless illness and nearly all have died within three years of onset. As such, this disease represents the most threatening of the acquired immunodeficiencies—a perturbation much more profound and lethal than any of the acquired immunodeficiencies that have been associated frequently with other virus infections, nutritional deficiencies, cancers, aging, fungus infections, persistent bacterial infections, autoimmune diseases, or endocrine disturbances.

The life-threatening nature of AIDS derives from the fact that this immunodeficiency is not only profound, but persistent and progressive. Once the immunodeficiency has been diagnosed, this disease has thus far been irreversible. In this way, it must be contrasted to SCID, in which cellular engineering, using bone marrow transplantation from a matched sibling, a matched relative, a partially matched relative, or a parental haploidentical donor can be curative. The latter approach involves a new method for administration of marrow after removal of the unwanted post thymic cells by lectin separation. With AIDS, however, even though one life-threatening opportunistic infection is recognized and treated successfully, another soon occurs. Ultimately, an infecting pathogen will erupt that cannot be coped with by the responsible physician even though he may be employing the most advanced forms of modern chemotherapeutics and antibiotics. Among the infections that occur in patients with AIDS are those caused by fungi, bacteria, viruses, and protozoa.

The list of organisms plaguing the patient with AIDS includes organisms that are normally resisted by mechanisms involving either cell-mediated immunities or antibodies or both, but it is particularly rich in the microorganisms against which the T cell–mediated immunities are known to be deployed (Table 1). As if this long list of opportunistic infections were not threat enough to these patients, they are also prone to develop malignant diseases. Listed on Table 2 are the malignancies that have already been encountered in these patients. It seems likely that the cancers that appear so soon after the onset of the immunodeficiency in these patients include some malignancies in which virus agents play a predominant role. Several patients with AIDS have developed lymphomas of the central nervous system. This

---

Table 1

Opportunistic Infections in Patients with AIDS

1. Herpes simplex	9. Toxoplasma
2. Cytomegalovirus	10. Pneumocystis
3. Varicella zoster virus	11. Mycobacterium TBC
4. Hepatitis B virus	12. Mycobacterium atypical
5. Adenovirus	13. Cryptosporidium
6. Epstein-Barr virus	14. Cryptococcus
7. Papovavirus	15. Candida
8. Legionella	

Table 2

Malignant Diseases Encountered in AIDS Patients

1. Kaposi's sarcoma
2. Non-Hodgkin's B cell lymphoma
3. Undifferentiated B cell lymphoma
4. Burkitt's lymphoma
5. Diffuse large cell B lymphoma
6. Hodgkin's disease
7. Squamous cell carcinoma

is important because it is a complication seen also in children with the Wiskott-Aldrich immunodeficiency syndrome, in patients immunosuppressed to facilitate organ transplantation, and in patients with other primary immunodeficiencies, e.g., ataxia telangiectasia. Whether other cancers that reflect deficiencies in immunologic surveillance will appear will only be revealed in time, if and when the opportunistic infections can be sufficiently well controlled to permit more prolonged survival and, thus, a latent period long enough to spawn other forms of cancer.

The Immune Systems

To permit an understanding of the profound acquired immunodeficiency that occurs in patients with AIDS, it is essential to describe briefly and in relatively simple terms the cells and cellular interactions now known to be involved in the immunological defenses. Figure 1 represents the basic two cellular arms of the specific immune systems. One of the crucial cell populations, the T cells, develops under the inducing and differentiative influence of the thymus. Precursor cells, which have been acted upon by thymic hormones, must traffic to the thymus, where they are induced to develop into cells that become T lymphocytes. Some of these cells that are then exported from the thymus are short-lived cells and some are long-lived. Thymus hormones may act on cells that have left the thymus to ensure their further development and maturation. Once these T lymphocytes have matured, they have the capacity to recognize differences between foreign cells and foreign antigens on the one hand, and self-cells and self-antigens on the other. These T lymphocytes are very mobile. They

FIGURE 1*

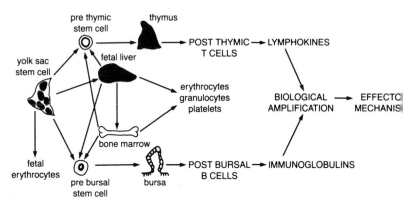

circulate through blood and lymph and then recirculate by leaving the blood or lymph to percolate through the tissues of the body, where they can detect substances like bacteria, fungi, protozoa, and virus-infected cells as being foreign. When they have detected such foreigners by cell-surface detector mechanisms, they are transformed into cells that divide and expand their numbers and begin to produce chemical messengers, called lymphokines, that can increase the function of phagocytic defense cells, induce inflammation, enhance vascular reactivity, and even alter the coagulation of the blood. After recognizing foreign antigens, they produce several of these lymphokines, which may act like hormones or growth factors to facilitate cell division and very much expand the numbers of immunologically active T lymphocytes by acting at the cell surface through receptors on the membrane of these cells. Factors produced by T cells of certain subpopulations can also act to promote the growth and development of the cells of an alternative line of development—the B lymphocytes. These T lymphocytes, working with other cells in the body, especially the macrophages, are crucial to the rejection of foreign cells and tissues and to the bodily defense against virus-infected cells, fungus-infected cells, and certain protozoa. By activating the macrophages, the T cells also stimulate the destruction of bacteria that have been engulfed by the phagocytes.

*Robert A. Good, "Organization and differentiation in the lymphoid system," in *Neonatal Hepatitis and Biliary Atresia*, N. B. Javitt (ed.), DHEW Publication No. (NIH) 79-1296 (Washington, D.C.: U.S. Government Printing Office, 1979), p. 91.

The alternative major arm of the immunity system is represented by the B lymphocytes. The B lymphocytes are a much more sessile cell population than the T lymphocytes, although a few of them also circulate in the peripheral blood and lymph. The B lymphocytes develop under a crucial influence that is different from that exercised by the thymus itself. B lymphocytes first appear in fetal liver, but later seem to be spawned in the bone marrow of mammals and man. In birds, they are developed in a thymuslike organ located at the tail end of the gastrointestinal tract and called the bursa of Fabricius. The name "B lymphocytes" reflects these cells' origins in either bursa or bone marrow. B lymphocytes are the precursors of the plasma cells, which are literally the factories of antibody and immunoglobulin production. The development of B lymphocytes into antibody-producing factories is strongly influenced by products of the T lymphocytes. The antibodies produced by the B lymphocytes enter the blood and lymph, where they can react with foreign antigens. Once this reaction has taken place, the complex formed between foreign antigen and antibody produced by the B lymphocyte can interact in a sequence or cascade with circulating proteins called complement proteins. These complement components are precursors of enzymes that, when activated, produce products that initiate inflammation, facilitate phagocytosis and lyse foreign cells and microorganisms, and destroy or neutralize viruses. The complement cascade amplifies, several thousandfold, the influence of certain antibodies on a molecule-for-molecule basis and thus amplifies greatly the immunologic influences of the B lymphocytes.

Similarly, the influence of T lymphocytes in the bodily defense on a cell-for-cell basis is amplified several thousandfold by their production or generation of biologically active molecules now called lymphokines, growth factors, and differentiation factors. Thus both T cells and B cells exert powerful influences in defending the body through their own products and also through their influence on the phagocytes, both microphages and macrophages, the inflammatory process, the reactions of blood vessels, and the coagulation of blood and lymph.

During the past fifteen years, intensive research has shown that the functions of these two major lymphocyte populations are greatly influenced, both positively and negatively, by each other and that the immunological systems represent systems that are highly regulated by the lymphoid cells themselves as well as by external influences such as those exercised by the brain or endocrine glands.

The autoregulation or self-regulation derives, in large part, from specialization of the lymphocytes into distinct subpopulations. These have been called helper or suppressor lymphocytes. Cells of the helper subpopulation are involved in facilitating the activation, differentiation, and function of both T and B lymphocytes. Cells of the suppressor subpopulation are capable of inhibiting B lymphocyte development to plasma cells and, thus, inhibiting antibody production. Now, with the development of a powerful new technology based on harnessing a super-antibody-producing plasma cell line that produces the so-called monoclonal antibodies, it has become possible to prepare antibodies that can be produced in factories, marketed, and thus made available as uniform products around the world. The monoclonal antibodies prepared against surface antigens of T lymphocytes have made it possible to distinguish T cells from B cells, to recognize the several stages in the development of normal T cells and B cells, and even to recognize each of the subpopulations of T lymphocytes and B lymphocytes from one another. With these powerful new tools, it has become possible to analyze more effectively than ever before the immunological abnormalities that underlie genetically determined immunodeficiencies and to analyze as well the perturbations of B cell and T cell development that occur in patients with acquired immunodeficiencies, including those with AIDS. Medical laboratories can do this uniformly because their immunological tests can be based on monoclonal antibodies that are identical or similar in every laboratory.

Table 3 lists some of the monoclonal antibodies, already marketed by two companies, that permit, in subpopulations of T lymphocytes, identification and quantification of the numbers of cells that can be recognized within the thymus, in the blood and lymph, and in the peripheral lymphoid tissue of humans. Normal values for lymphocytes, as well as for numbers of cells of each of these subpopulations, have

Table 3

Ortho Laboratories		*Becton-Dickinson*
OKT 3	All T cells	Leu-1 Leu-4
OKT 11	E rosette receptor (T cells)	Leu-5
OKT 4	Helper T cell subpopulation	Leu-3
OKT 5	Suppressor cytotoxic	Leu-2A
OKT 8	T cell subpopulation	Leu-2B
OKT 6	Thymus lymphocyte	Leu-6
OKT 7	Natural killer cell	Leu-7

been established for persons of all age groups so that disturbances that occur with disease can be recognized, as can consequences of pharmacological and cellular manipulations carried out in an effort to correct immunodeficiencies.

The Natural Killer Cells

Relatively recently, a new population of lymphoid cells has been recognized that circulates in the blood, lymph nodes, spleen, and other lymphoid tissues. These cells are called natural killer (NK) cells. They are capable of recognizing, as foreign, tumor cells, virus-infected cells, and even embryonic cells that are out of place. The NK cells can initiate chemical processes that destroy these cells and initiate their elimination from the body. Tissue culture methods have been developed to assess the functions of the NK cells, and monoclonal antibodies have been developed that permit their identification and quantitative enumeration. These NK cells may contain populations of the cells that are of paramount importance in surveillance against cancer and virus-infected cells. When the NK cells are absent or deficient, as they are in certain rare patients who have a genetically determined inborn error, the patients are especially prone to develop lymphoid malignancies and virus infection. The NK cells are important in an additional way. They are activated and/or increased in number by the influences of interferon. These cells, as well as the T lymphocytes and B lymphocytes, seem to be very much involved in the immunodeficiency seen in patients with AIDS.

Thus, we can no longer think of simply two arms of the immunity system subserving antibody production on the one hand and cellular immunities on the other, but must consider the immunity systems as complex interacting populations of lymphocytes that facilitate and modulate one another in complex ways. It appears as though the arms have hands and fingers that work together to make it possible for humans to maintain their integrity as individuals in that sea of bacteria, fungi, protozoa, and viruses in which we all live (Figure 2). This system also seems to be finely tuned to recognize changes in the body's cells that occur when a virus invades the cell, or to recognize changes that are associated with the development of malignant characteristics. Thus, when the immunity systems are deficient or abnormal, increased susceptibility to infection, propensity to autoimmunity, and increase in certain tumors is a regular concomitant.

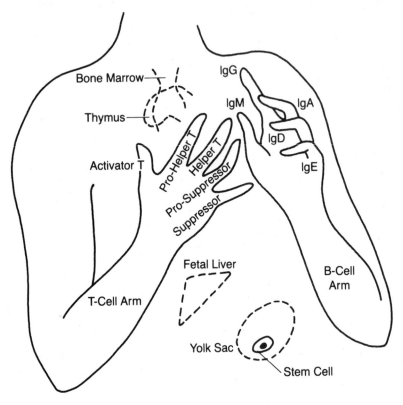

FIGURE 2
The Two Arms of the Specific Immunity System

The Immunologic Abnormality in AIDS

It is the appearance of perturbations of these beautiful means of the bodily defense that looms as the central issue in AIDS. Table 4 lists the major immunodeficiencies that have been identified in patients with AIDS. These include anergy to skin test antigens that elicit a high frequency of delayed allergy in healthy members of the general population. The total lymphocyte count is low, the number of T lymphocytes is very much reduced, and lymphocyte functions are drastically deficient. With respect to delayed allergic responses, however, it is important to realize that, at least early in the course of AIDS,

Table 4
Immunodeficiency in AIDS

1. Cutaneous anergy
   a. delayed allergy to common antigens usually deficient
   b. 2-4 DNCB sensitizability absent
   c. recall delayed allergy absent late but not early
2. Proliferative responses of lymphocytes deficient
   a. PHA—low—progressive decline
   b. Con A—low—progressive decline
   c. PWM—low—but more variable
   d. common antigens—low—progressive decline
3. Reduced numbers of lymphocytes
4. Reduced numbers of T lymphocytes
5. Net decrease of T helper cells (T_4-Leu 3)
6. Conservation of T suppressor cells (T_{5-8}-Leu 2) normal or slightly low
7. Suppressor cells not spontaneously activated
8. NK cells may be normal, slightly depressed or severely depressed, often defects in NK activity
9. Circulating levels of interferon normal
10. Capacity to produce alpha-interferon OK

recall-delayed allergy may remain normal, even in patients with severe AIDS, as Dr. Fred Siegal has reported. The sensitizability of these patients to 2-4-dinitrochlorobenzene, however, seems regularly to be grossly deficient.

Profound, Persistent, and Progressive Immunodeficiency

In patients with AIDS, the immunodeficiency is progressive, and as the patients develop opportunistic infections, the immunodeficiency proves to be profound, persistent, and progressive. On Table 5 are listed the abnormalities in the proliferative responses of the lymphocytes that have been revealed in the studies of Drs. Susanna Cunningham-Rundles, Thomas Spiro, and several others. The proliferative responses to phytohemagglutinin (PHA), concanavalin A (Con A), and pokeweed mitogen are all low, and those to PHA and Con A, which represent proliferative responses of the T lymphocytes, are particularly low and are prone to show a progressive decline. Responses to pokeweed mitogen, which is a T cell–dependent B cell proliferation,

Table 5

Immunologic Abnormality in AIDS

1. Absolute numbers of lymphocytes regularly low
2. Absolute number of T_4-Leu 3 populations very low
3. Absolute number of helper/inducer T_{5-8} or Leu 2 low but less depressed than B
4. Ratio of B/C very low—regularly inverted

are more variable and likely not to show such a steep progressive decline. Proliferative responses to common antigens like staphylococci, candida, and coloform organisms are regularly low and show a progressive decline with persistent disease. Recently Susanna Cunningham-Rundles and her colleagues have found that serum of patients with AIDS will inhibit proliferative responses of normal lymphocytes to the common antigens and phytomitogens.

Lymphocytes in AIDS

The abnormalities of lymphocyte numbers is one of the most consistent abnormalities in AIDS. The absolute number of lymphocytes is always low by the time AIDS is recognized. In addition, the number of cells in the subpopulation of T lymphocytes recognized by monoclonal antibodies that define the T helper cells is regularly extremely low. Indeed, the decrease in the numbers of these helper cells is even more extreme than the depression of total T cells. By contrast, the absolute number of T lymphocytes of the suppressor phenotype, although somewhat low, is better preserved. Thus, the helper T lymphocyte/suppressor T lymphocyte ratio is inverted and exceedingly low when these ratios are compared to almost any other disease (Table 5). Everyone who has studied the lymphocyte number in patients with AIDS has made this same observation, as this abnormality is consistent in patients with AIDS. There is, however, no evidence that the suppressor population of T lymphocytes has been activated in patients with this disease.

The numbers of NK cells and NK function in the patients with AIDS thus far reported has been quite variable. In most instances, the kind of NK cells that have the capacity to destroy virus-infected cells is very much decreased, but some patients with AIDS have had normal NK function as measured with other target cells. Similarly, the numbers and functions of NK cells that can spontaneously kill tumor cells, such as the K562 erythroleukemia line, are usually, but not always, decreased. The number of large granular lymphocytes bearing the definitive cell-surface marker antigens is usually very low in patients with this disease. The level of interferon, which has the capacity to augment function of the NK cells, is often depressed in patients with AIDS who suffer from Kaposi's sarcoma and in those with the generalized adenitis syndrome associated with one of the earliest manifestations of AIDS. NK cell function and numbers, by contrast, are usually quite normal in homosexual controls.

Ability to produce interferon of the alpha type seems to be quite normal in most patients with AIDS, but it is also occasionally depressed in these patients. Again, Dr. S. Cunningham-Rundles has studied the influence of serum from patients with AIDS and found that some of the sera blocked interferon-induced NK activity, but not endogenous NK activity.

Autologous Mixed Leukocyte Reaction

Another potentially very important interaction of lymphoid cells appears to be disturbed in patients with AIDS. When one analyzes the capacity of non-T lymphocytes to stimulate T lymphocytes to proliferate in patients with AIDS and those with AIDS who suffer from Kaposi's sarcoma, the autologous mixed lymphocyte reaction is depressed, as was shown by Gupta and Safai. Further, non-T lymphocytes of patients with AIDS are poor stimulators, and the T cells of patients with AIDS are poor responders in allogeneic mixed leukocyte reactions (Table 6).

Table 6
Immunodeficiency in AIDS—Mixed Leukocyte Reactions

1. Autologous mixed lymphocyte reaction depressed
2. Allogeneic mixed lymphocyte reaction depressed
3. Non-T cells poor stimulators in allogeneic MLR
4. T cells poor responders in allogeneic MLR

The Association with the DR-5 Antigen in Patients with AIDS

A few years ago, it was first observed that a high proportion of Americans and Europeans with classical Kaposi's sarcoma express the DR-5 antigen on their lymphocytes. The DR antigens seem to play important roles in determining the magnitude of specific immune responses to particular antigens. The genetic determinants for these antigens are located in the polymorphic immune response-gene section of the major histocompatibility complex located on chromosome #6 in humans. The genes of the histocompatibility complex are crucial to the identification of a person's immunological individuality. Specifically, these genes play important roles in defense against virus-infected cells and cooperation of lymphocytes in immune responses, thus determining the magnitude of antibody responses as well as determining the antigenicity of a person's tissue, on which graft rejections are based. It thus seemed especially important when the Kaposi's sarcoma associated with AIDS was discovered by Pablo Rubenstein and his colleagues (as well as DuPont and his colleagues) to be also linked to the DR-5 determinant. It now seems of greatest importance to know whether the forms of Kaposi's sarcoma that occur in hemophiliacs, Haitian immigrants, and African patients with AIDS are associated with DR-5. It also seems extremely important to know if the invasive form of Kaposi's sarcoma that occurs so frequently in young East African blacks has an intimate association with the operation of the DR-5 antigen coded for in the MHR of chromosome #6.

Disturbances of B Lymphocytes in Patients with AIDS

The consistent deficiencies of helper T cell subpopulations, the cell-mediated immune functions, as well as the inordinate susceptibility to infection with viruses, fungi, and protozoa, have made most immunologists who have studied patients with the AID syndrome accept the view that disturbances of T cell numbers and functions are the primary and thus the critically immunologic abnormality in patients with AIDS. However, Dr. Susan Zolla-Pazner has emphasized the B cell abnormalities in patients with AIDS and has proposed that the B cell abnormalities in this disease may be as crucial as they are in patients with infectious mononucleosis and as the complex syndrome of profound immunodeficiency defined by David Purtillo is in patients who cannot defend themselves against the Epstein-Barr (EB) virus. The B cell abnormalities identified and emphasized by Dr.

Susan Zolla-Pazner in patients with AIDS include the following: abundant mitotic activity of B lymphocytes; plasmacytosis in lymphoid tissue and bone marrow; abundant germinal follicles in spleen and lymph nodes; excessive number of lymphoblasts in the blood and lymphoid tissues. All of these are hallmarks of increased B lymphocyte activity. Further, high levels of each of the immunoglobulins are usually found in the blood of patients with AIDS, and high levels of antibodies, including many autoantibodies, reflect what must be an excessive polyclonal activation of B lymphocytes in patients with AIDS. Levels in the circulating blood of B2 microglobulin, a membrane component of the B cells closely linked chemically to antibody molecules, are also exceedingly high in patients with AIDS who have infections with *Pneumocystis carinii*, cytomegalovirus, and *Mycobacterium avium*. This finding suggests that there is an increased proliferation and turnover of B lymphocytes in patients with AIDS.

In addition to these evidences of excessive B cell proliferation and activation, the lymph nodes of patients with AIDS show evidence of excessive capillary proliferation, necrosis, and granuloma formation. These changes are often seen in other circumstances when B cell activation is excessive, for example, following extreme stimulation with antigens in patients with angioimmunoblastic lymphadenopathy, and are seen in the lymphoid tissues of certain strains of autoimmune mice.

Reflecting the immunological excesses on the B cell side of immunity in patients with AIDS, levels of circulating immune complexes, antigens, antibodies or immunoglobulins and complement have also been found to be markedly elevated in some patients with AIDS and significantly elevated in most. Autoantibodies are also frequently present in the blood of patients with AIDS, and these have included antibodies directed toward neutrophils, platelets, or even toward T lymphocytes. Studies still urgently needed are measurements of autoantibodies directed toward antigens on the T_4-Leu 2 subpopulation of lymphocytes, which is so much depressed in patients with AIDS.

Thymus Hormone Levels

Dr. Allan Goldstein of George Washington University has developed a radioimmunoassay that permits quantitation of levels of at least one thymic hormone, thymosin alpha-1. Circulating levels of this hormone have been reported to be markedly elevated in patients with AIDS. In this way, AIDS patients are like certain patients suffering from cancers associated with defective immune responses who may also have high levels of thymic hormone. Also to be considered in this context are the very high levels of thymic hormonelike activity, which Dr. Bijan Safai and I discovered in patients with mycosis fungoides, even very late in life when the thymus is usually very atrophic. Perhaps thymosin alpha-1 as well as thymopoietinlike activity and facteur thymique serique activity can be generated in sites other than the thymus under pathological conditions such as AIDS. This seems to be another indication that there is a serious dysregulation of immune functions in patients with AIDS, which is quite surprising in the face of observations that indicate paradoxically that the thymus at postmortem is severely involuted in many of the patients with AIDS, who are young and normally should have a large, active thymus.

Depressed Helper/Suppressor Ratios in Other Diseases

Listed in Table 7 are several other diseases that have already been associated with depressed ratios of the helper/suppressor T cell subpopulations. It will be seen in the table that this list of diseases includes diseases in which patients suffer from persistent infections as well as certain transient virus infections. In addition, this abnormality of immune cell numbers is also seen in promiscuous homosexuals who are known to experience many sexually transmitted infections and in hemophiliacs who have been treated with injections of concentrates of the antihemophiliac Factor VIII. However, the immunodeficiency and

---

Table 7

Diseases Sometimes Associated with Disturbance of T Cell Subpopulations and/or Deficiencies of Delayed Allergy

1. Measles—rubeola
2. German measles—rubella
3. Influenza
4. Hepatitis B
5. Cancers
   a. Hodgkin's disease
   b. head and neck epitheliomas
   c. colon cancer
   d. breast cancer
   e. others
6. Autoimmunities
7. Leprosy

---

immunologic perturbation in AIDS is generally more profound, more progressive, and more persistent than is seen in any of these other diseases.

The Immunological Abnormality of Homosexuals

Disturbances of immunological functions are very frequent among homosexual males. These persons, especially those who are promiscuous, have a high frequency of venereal infection. They also have a high frequency of immunological abnormality. However, in almost all instances, the immunological abnormality is very different from that observed in patients with AIDS with opportunistic infections, Kaposi's sarcoma, or the profound lymphadenopathic abnormality. In healthy homosexuals who do not suffer from AIDS, the T cell number is usually not decreased. The total number of cells of the helper-containing subpopulation T_4-Leu 3 is not decreased. The number of lymphocytes in the T_{5-8}-Leu 2 population that contains the bulk of suppressor T lymphocytes is relatively and often absolutely elevated, and the suppressor cell functional potential is also increased (Table 8).

Table 8
Healthy Homosexuals

1. T cell number not decreased
2. T_4-Leu 3 population not decreased
3. T_{5-8}-Leu 2 population relatively and usually absolutely high
4. Suppressor functional potential increased

The Immunological Abnormality of Hemophiliacs

Hemophiliacs who have been treated with Factor VIII concentrate but not those treated with cryoprecipitate have developed AIDS. Indeed, already the incidence of AIDS, either with or without Kaposi's sarcoma, in the hemophiliacs treated with Factor VIII concentrate is higher than in homosexuals; it has reached approximately 1/1,000. When it occurs in the hemophiliacs, AIDS has been associated with the same immunologic and cellular abnormalities that have been observed in the intravenous drug users, male homosexuals, and Haitians who have developed this disease. The essential abnormalities observed include evidence of polyclonal B cell activation coupled with regular severe selective T helper cell deficiency, inability to express delayed allergic responses, and frequent NK cell deficiency and malfunction.

However, the population of hemophiliacs who develop AIDS represents only a tiny proportion of the hemophiliacs who have been treated with Factor VIII containing lyophilized concentrate of pooled plasma. As a group, these as yet healthy hemophiliacs also show evidence of immunological perturbation. Like the healthy homosexuals, the hemophiliacs treated in this way have unusually high numbers of the suppressor population and consequently have inverted ratios of the helper/suppressor T cells. Whether or not persons in this population of hemophiliacs are at risk of developing AIDS is not yet clear, but thus far, patients having the abnormality of lymphoid cell population have not been shown to progress into fully expressed AIDS.

In the few cases where AIDS has apparently been transferred by blood transfusion, the immunological disturbances that have occurred have been identical to those of the AIDS with or without Kaposi's sarcoma.

Renal Transplant Recipients

Kaposi's sarcoma was shown several years ago to occur with inordinate frequency along with lymphomas and certain other cancers—especially B cell and Burkitt's lymphomas—in renal transplant patients. The Kaposi's sarcoma observed in the renal transplant recipient has regularly been associated with evidence of persistent infection with cytomegalovirus (CMV). Likewise, the B cell lymphomas and Burkitt's lymphomas have been associated with virological and serological evidence of persistent EB virus infection. Immunological abnormalities and immunodysregulation have regularly been present in these patients. Indeed, their immunologic abnormalities are usually identical to those seen in male homosexuals with AIDS. Like homosexuals with AIDS, the renal transplant patients with Kaposi's sarcoma have decreased numbers of T cells, markedly decreased T_4 helper lymphocytes, decreased T_{5-8} suppressor cells, and an extremely low or reversed T_4/T_{5-8} helper/suppressor cell ratio (Table 9).

In this disease, it seems to be chemical plus hormonal immunosuppression that opens the door to the development of a life-threatening immunodysregulation that, in turn, predisposes to opportunistic infec-

Table 9
Renal Transplant Recipients

Kaposi's sarcoma
CMV infection frequent
T cells decreased
T_4-Leu 3 ↓↓↓
T_{5-8}-Leu 2 depressed, normal, or slightly depressed
Immunosuppression with chemicals and hormones opens the door

tion and Kaposi's sarcoma. It is encouraging to note that when immunosuppressive treatment of these patients is removed, the Kaposi's sarcoma as well as the profound persistent immunodeficiency undergoes regression. These findings urge continued intensive study of patients with AIDS in hopes of finding a simple means of correcting their life-threatening immunodeficiency.

Kaposi's Sarcoma in Africa

Kaposi's sarcoma as it occurs among young males, especially in equatorial East Africa, can, as other forms of Kaposi's sarcoma, be shown regularly to be associated with persistent infection with the CMV. This form of Kaposi's sarcoma differs from other forms of Kaposi's sarcoma in that it is invasive and may be very extensive. Deficiencies of cell-mediated immunities have been observed in these patients and T cell numbers are often decreased. However, definitive studies of numbers of cells in each of the T cell subpopulations and ratios of T_4 helper/T_{5-8} suppressor populations have not yet been presented for this group of patients. These patients, like those with AIDS, may succumb to intercurrent infections, but in East Africa, as Templeton has pointed out, it is malaria, filariasis, typhoid fever, and salmonellosis that present the greatest burden of infection instead of the long list of unusual opportunistic infections that occur in patients with Kaposi's sarcoma associated with AIDS.

Whether epidemic Kaposi's sarcoma of equatorial Africa is related to AIDS is not clear, but recent studies from Belgium and France have discerned black patients with classical AIDS without Kaposi's sarcoma. In these patients, the immunodeficiency includes the immunologic dysregulations and helper/suppressor subpopulation abnormality described above. Only additional studies will ascertain the relationships between these African cases of AIDS, the characteristic fulminant and invasive Kaposi's sarcoma of equatorial Africa, and AIDS in European and American homosexuals and the Haitian heterosexuals. Nonetheless, the gross immunologic abnormalities appear to be similar in all of these groups. However, definitive analysis of the immunological perturbations in African patients with Kaposi's sarcoma, using modern technology, seems urgently needed at this writing. Similarly, it seems especially important to ascertain whether African blacks with Kaposi's sarcoma, with or without the persistent, profound, and progressive immunodeficiency, have Kaposi's sarcoma in association with the presence of DR-5 antigen determined in the genes of the major histocompatibility complex.

Immunodeficiencies and CMV Infection

Since CMV infection can be associated with all forms of Kaposi's sarcoma thus far studied, and since Kaposi's sarcoma occurs in high frequency in male homosexuals with AIDS, it is particularly important to know whether the immunodysregulation so typical of AIDS is found in other patients with CMV infection. The answer is usually negative. CMV produces a form of infectious mononucleosis. Analyses of lymphocyte function and lymphocyte subpopulations have been made in this disease. As with other viral infections, including rubeola, influenza, and rubella, CMV infection sometimes produces immunosuppressive effects. However, as in each of the other viral infections, the immunodeficiency has been transient and has not led to the persistent, profound, and progressive immunodeficiency and immunological dysregulation that occurs in patients with AIDS. However, studies must be made of the highly lethal persistent form of CMV infection that occurs in neonates and is sometimes seen in other forms in children who are immunodeficient.

Summary

Patients with AIDS, whether associated with Kaposi's sarcoma or recurrent life-threatening opportunistic infection or with severe lymphadenopathy and night sweating, have a profound deficiency of immunological functions and characteristic evidence of severe immunodysregulation. The abnormalities of immunologic function include evidence of profound T helper set deficiencies, deficient cell-mediated immunities, and frequent deficiencies of certain NK functions. The ratio of T_4-Leu 3 helper cells to T_{5-8}-Leu 2 suppressor cells is regularly dramatically decreased, and the total number of T cells are usually markedly decreased. These findings are not characteristic of healthy homosexuals or healthy hemophiliacs who may have immunological abnormalities. The latter often have increased numbers of the suppressor-cytotoxic T_{5-8}-Leu 2 lymphocyte subset and, consequently, inverted ratios of lympho helper/suppressor subsets. *In vitro* responses of T lymphocytes to phytomitogens and common antigens are greatly depressed in the classical AIDS and are much less depressed or perfectly normal in the healthy hemophiliacs and healthy homosexuals.

The B cell numbers and functions are also regularly perturbed in patients with AIDS showing evidence of excessive stimulation and proliferation of B cells, polyclonal B cell activation, and increased B2 microglobulin levels. These abnormalities are reflected in the increased circulatory levels of all of the immunoglobulins coupled with decreased *in vitro* responses to specific antigens.

The challenge before modern immunologists will be to show, as a consequence of their analyses, that they can find means to restore the immunologic functions of patients with AIDS to normal and to stop the carnage that is consequent to the increased susceptibility to opportunistic infections in this disease. This is a challenge that has not yet been met, and represents a big order. It is, however, a challenge worthy of the surging knowledge of the immunologic system and the increasing understanding of the control of lymphocyte function. The approach can take momentum from the progressively successful manipulation of these complex relationships in the repeatedly successful correction of the immunological abnormalities in lethal, severe, congenital immunodeficiencies like SCID and the Wiskott-Aldrich syndrome. It is certain, however, that if AIDS can be corrected by measures of cellular engineering, we will know much more about the immunological functions, the relation of the immunological systems and cells to one another, and also more about the regulation of immunity than we know right now. I am sure, however, that the ingenuity is at hand in the immunological community to remove the pall of death that at the moment attends this awful epidemic.

Part III

The Clinical
Picture

If one views medicine as an ongoing battle, then the clinician is the point man. He is the doctor tending the sick patient. He supplies the vital information to the epidemiologist and must translate the findings of the laboratory research scientist into a specific treatment for individual patients. Here four clinicians discuss the signs, symptoms, and therapy of AIDS patients.

Dr. Donald Armstrong, Chief of Infectious Diseases at Memorial Sloan-Kettering Cancer Center in New York City, has had vast experience with viral disorders in patients receiving anti-cancer drugs that often damage the immune system. He, therefore, brings to the problem of AIDS an unusual understanding of the pattern of viral diseases in the immune-compromised patient.

Dr. Donald Louria, Professor of Public Health at the University of New Jersey College of Medicine, is widely known for his skill in the management of complex fungal and bacterial infections. His paper provides another perspective on the many-faceted clinical picture presented by AIDS.

My own involvement with AIDS patients stems from the frequency of parasitic diseases among homosexual men and from the growing realization that parasites are, by far, the most common cause of death in fatal cases of AIDS. In my chapter, I consider the management of overwhelming parasitic infections, including the difficult decisions in balancing the dangers and benefits of highly toxic drugs.

A frequent manifestation of AIDS is a type of cancer formerly considered extremely rare. No one has seen more of this cancer than Dr. Bijan Safai, Chief of Dermatology at Memorial Sloan-Kettering in New York City, who shares with us his expertise on Kaposi's sarcoma.

5

Viral Infections

Donald Armstrong, M.D.

The Acquired Immune Deficiency Syndrome is a devastating disease, probably of viral origin, that renders people susceptible to a number of viral, as well as other, opportunistic infections and neoplasms. Even the neoplasms may well be caused by viruses.

Etiology of AIDS

The epidemiology of AIDS strongly implicates an infectious agent as the cause. The agent is transmitted by 1) male-to-male sexual contact, 2) exchange of blood, 3) unknown means among the Haitians, 4) Factor VIII concentrate from multiple donors, and 5) close contact between parent and child in the home. It may be spread by 6) male-to-female sexual contact, and 7) infusion of blood products from single as well as multiple donors. In the first four situations there are enough cases to convince most workers in the field that this is a proven method of transmission.

The case for male-to-female transmission is not entirely convincing. There is one instance where a woman who lived with an intravenous drug abuser developed AIDS, while other women in similar situations have developed T lymphocyte immunological abnormalities as demonstrated by laboratory tests. We have to accept the word of these women that they were not intravenous drug abusers themselves to accept this evidence. Many of us do not. Similarly, the cases reported following blood product administration are few and it is possible that other factors might have made these people immunodeficient. In either of these situations, if this is a method of transmission, we should see more cases, which will finally convince the skeptics.

Accepting just the first five modes of transmission, the agent demonstrates definite characteristics. It is transmitted in a similar manner to hepatitis B virus (HBV), cytomegalovirus (CMV), Epstein-Barr virus (EBV), and perhaps hepatitis non-A, non-B virus (H non-A, BV). By serological testing, our studies on non-Haitians with Kaposi's sarcoma (KS) and opportunistic infections (OI) show that almost 100 percent of patients with AIDS have evidence of infection with all of the above viruses for which we have tests. Other viruses that are believed by many to be candidates are delta virus, parvoviruses, polyoma viruses, adenoviruses, and arboviruses.

It is possible that a non-viral agent, transmitted in a similar fashion to those viruses mentioned above, is responsible. Frequently in the history of medicine, disease has been attributed to a virus that later proved to be due to another type of infectious agent. Recent and excellent examples are atypical pneumonias that were proved to be caused by *Mycoplasma pneumoniae*; Legionnaires' disease, which is due to fastidious bacteria, the *Legionella* species; and Lyme disease, now demonstrated to be caused by a spirochete. Nonetheless, I would suggest that a virus is more likely to be found as the cause of AIDS because viruses have been clearly demonstrated to be capable of causing T lymphocyte immunodeficiencies in man and animals (e.g., CMV) and also that they are capable of inducing transformation and neoplasms in cell cultures (EBV), in animals (retroviruses), and probably in man (EBV).

There are arguments for and against each of the candidate viruses and there may be an undescribed virus responsible. The documentation of this virus is crucial to establishing the epidemiology of this disease so that preventive measures can be instituted and so that the origin and development of the immune defect can be understood and measures developed to correct it.

Viral-Symptomatic Diseases in AIDS

Table 1

Viruses Responsible for Symptomatic Infection in AIDS

Virus	*Syndromes*
Cytomegalovirus	Pneumonia
	Colitis
	Retinitis
	Encephalitis
	Disseminated
	? Kaposi's sarcoma
Herpes simplex II	Progressive ulcers
	Colitis
	Disseminated
Varicella-zoster virus	Herpes zoster—prolonged
	Herpes zoster—disseminated
Epstein-Barr virus	? Burkitt's lymphoma
	? B cell lymphomas
Hepatitis B virus	Chronic active hepatitis
Hepatitis A virus	Acute hepatitis
Adenovirus	Colonized
	Disseminated
Papovaviruses	Progressive multifocal
	Leucoencephalopathy

Cytomegalovirus

By serologic tests, almost every patient with AIDS whom we have studied has antibody to CMV. Infection, then, is consistent, but disease occurs less regularly. Symptomatic CMV infection, however, is one of the most common that we and others have documented in AIDS patients, following only *Pneumocystis carinii* pneumonia (PCP) and herpes simplex virus (HSV) infections. Cytomegalovirus infections are more difficult to document than PCP and HSV infection and are probably more common than recorded. Invasive infection with CMV is often appreciated only at postmortem examination. Even then it may be difficult to fully correlate the histopathology with a CMV isolate that could reflect an unrelated viremia.

Disseminated CMV infection with involvement of multiple organs is manifested primarily by fever, weight loss, and liver function abnormalities. After weeks to months of such symptoms a patient may then go on to develop pneumonia or colitis. The pneumonia may be due to CMV alone, but it is often mixed with PCP. Likewise, the colitis may be due to CMV alone, but may also be mixed with herpes simplex. *Mycobacterium avium-intracellulare* have been found causing disease along with CMV in the same gastrointestinal tract, and the same will probably be found for cryptosporidia.

There is usually nothing unique in CMV liver disease. Moderate elevations of both the SGOT (4 to 8× normal) and the alkaline phosphatase (2 to 3× normal) are common. A liver biopsy showing cells typical of cytomegalic disease is necessary to confirm the diagnosis in addition to a positive culture. Occasionally only lymphocytic infiltration, without typical cytomegalic cells but with positive cultures, is seen; this probably represents true CMV disease. Studies for virus antigen and genomes in liver cells, macrophages, and lymphocytes should be done to document disease due to the CMV that is isolated in cell culture. Pneumonias also usually require a biopsy for diagnosis. The most reliable is an open lung biopsy, but a transbronchial biopsy has been adequate in some cases to show the cells with typical cytomegalic inclusions. A bronchoalveolar lavage alone may reveal typical intranuclear inclusions in cells on cytologic examination. Just as with liver biopsies, CMV may be isolated from the lung in the absence of typical histopathology; it is still not clear how to interpret this. There is no effective treatment for cytomegalovirus pneumonia.

Cytomegalovirus colitis also requires biopsy for diagnosis. Again the typical cells with "owls-eye" inclusions should be seen, along with a positive culture. On endoscopy ulcers may be seen in the mucosa of the large bowel but there is nothing distinctive about them. There is no proven effective treatment for CMV colitis. Other treatable causes or concomitant infections such as amebae or chlamydiae should be ruled out.

Cytomegalovirus retinitis may be seen without other evidence of CMV infection. This syndrome has been well described in patients following renal and bone marrow transplantation and is now appearing in AIDS patients. The diagnosis is a clinical one that has usually been confirmed at autopsy. Large hemorrhages and white exudates within the retina are widespread and may involve the macula, resulting in impairment of vision that can progress to blindness. Sheathing of vessels is also seen. Retinitis due to CMV has been treated with high doses of Ara A (10 to 15 mg/kg/day) and there have been cases where some resolution of the retinitis occurred during therapy. There are two reservations about this type of therapy: first, the possibility of danger-

Table 2
Treatment of Viral Infection

Herpes simplex skin lesions	Acyclovir
Cytomegalovirus retinitis	Ara A
Progressive multifocal leukoencephalopathy	Ara C
Disseminated varicella-zoster	Ara A, FIAC
Hepatitis B	Interferon

ous bone marrow suppression in patients who regularly have poor marrow reserve, and second, the theoretical possibility of making the CMV worse by immunosuppression with Ara A and even inducing dissemination. We have observed AIDS cases where dissemination of CMV has occurred while patients were receiving an anti-herpes virus drug, 2'-fluoro-5-iodo-beta-D-arabinofuranoscylcytosine (FIAC), and we are concerned that this could occur with other similar drugs such as Ara A or acyclovir. It is important to rule out other more treatable causes of retinitis such as toxoplasmosis. A vitreous aspiration can be done to document the etiology because many of the AIDS patients will not develop a rise in antibody titers. If there is any doubt on clinical or laboratory grounds, empiric therapy for toxoplasmosis is appropriate.

Encephalitis may occur as part of the disseminated CMV syndrome, which involves liver, lungs, heart, pancreas, adrenals, brain—almost any organ can be seeded and invasively infected with CMV. Death is usually due to pneumonia, although CNS or hepatic failure can also occur.

Kaposi's sarcoma has also been associated with CMV infection, not only by finding higher titers of antibody in patients with classical KS, but also by showing CMV antigen or specific CMV genome DNA in KS biopsy or tissue culture specimens. These are preliminary findings and require further substantiation, but are most interesting.

Herpes Simplex Virus

The second most common symptomatic viral infection in patients with AIDS is perineal herpes—usually due to type II herpes simplex. In homosexual men, it is often seen as a perianal ulcer that is persistent and intermittently progressive to the point of severe, painful, debilitating ulceration reaching as much as twelve centimeters in diameter.

Such severe lesions have been treated with acyclovir, Ara A, and FIAC with prompt responses. Cultures became negative and ulcers healed. In some cases, they recur and require further treatment. In women similar severe perineal ulcers have occurred. Severe facial lesions that required and responded to acyclovir therapy have also been reported.

Herpes simplex was isolated at autopsy from multiple internal organs of one patient who had no skin lesions.

Varicella-Zoster Virus

Herpes zoster has appeared in patients with AIDS and has been described as especially severe and protracted. Widespread dissemination has been noted, but a benign course has also been observed. Whether treatment will be necessary remains to be seen. The treatment would be Ara A or FIAC.

Epstein-Barr Virus

Some of the lymphomas seen in patients with KS or OI have been particularly severe B cell lymphomas. Whether these are associated with EB virus remains to be proven. That association has been made in non-AIDS patients and it is suggested that it will be made here also. Diagnosis of recent or previous infection can be made serologically. An IgM and IgG antibody test can be done. EBV in lymphoma cells is demonstrated by growing the cells in culture and showing the presence of the virus in the cells by fluorescent antibody techniques. There is no treatment for severe EBV infections.

Hepatitis B Virus

Almost every patient with AIDS who has been studied has shown evidence of hepatitis B virus infection, usually by the presence of antibody.

Studies for the presence or absence of delta viruses or antibodies are in progress.

Chronic active or persistent hepatitis can occur in patients with AIDS but there is no evidence that it occurs more often than in the general population. Diagnosis of hepatitis B virus infection is made by demonstrating antigen or antibody in the serum. The presence of core or E antigen suggests recent acute infection while surface Ag can be found in chronic infections. There is no proven effective treatment for hepatitis B virus infections, although combinations of interferon and Ara A have been tried in chronic active hepatitis with some promising results.

Hepatitis A Virus

Antibody to hepatitis A virus has been found regularly in patients with AIDS. Clinical hepatitis seems no more severe than in general. Diagnosis is by antibody determination of IgM and IgG antibody, and there is no treatment at present.

Adenovirus

In our experience, adenovirus in patients with AIDS is remarkable in two ways: it is most frequently isolated from urine rather than from throat or stool, and it is of a higher serotype (34/35) than that normally found in throats and stools. These particular characteristics of the adenovirus are found, as far as we know, in only one other group of patients—those who have been immunosuppressed following bone marrow transplantation.

The isolates from the AIDS patients are usually from superficial sites and are not evidently responsible for disease. There have been cases of disease due to disseminated adenovirus infection in bone marrow transplant patients, and we assume we will see them in AIDS patients in the future. We have isolated the virus from the kidney of one AIDS patient at autopsy. Diagnosis of invasive disease is accomplished by biopsy and culture of an otherwise sterile organ.

There is no treatment for adenovirus infections.

Polyoma Viruses

Papovaviruses can cause papillomas and warts in patients with AIDS but not apparently worse than in a comparable general population (e.g., homosexuals seen in an STD clinic). Progressive multifocal leukoencephalopathy (PML) due to a wart type or papovaviruses is one of the more common central nervous system infections in these patients. The virus is apparently ubiquitous in that the majority of people tested have antibody. In immunosuppressed patients, such as those undergoing organ transplantation, the virus may be isolated from the urine without being responsible for actual illness. Disease is clinically manifest by loss of memory, inability to concentrate, and diffuse and focal neurological signs that wax and wane but are ultimately progressive to the point of diffuse motor weakness, depression, and inanition.

A computerized axial tomography (CAT) scan shows streaking and focal areas of decreased uptake due to loss of white matter, but the only specific means of diagnosis is brain biopsy. The biopsy shows a typical pattern on histopathology, with patches of demyelination and cells (oligodendrocytes) showing enlarged nuclei with inclusions around the patches. Electromicroscopy reveals sheets of typical viral particles, and special culture techniques may result in isolation of the virus. A DNA inhibitor, Ara C, has been used in the treatment of PML with some transient responses. Patients with AIDS have shown a similar syndrome without focal signs and at biopsy or autopsy a diffuse loss of white matter without evident virus particles. Cultures have been negative. Whether this is a viral disease remains to be proven.

Other Viral Infections

Extensive molluscum contagiosum due to the large pox virus has been noted in AIDS patients, but invasive disease has not been recorded.

AIDS patients must be investigated for undescribed viruses using unusual techniques such as co-cultivation of potentially infected cells with the target diagnostic cell and including techniques to fuse the cells to allow passage of highly cell-associated viruses. Cultivation of possibly infected cells such as T lymphocytes or their precursors should be done because those may be the cells infected with the etiologic agent, and the only way to prove this thesis would be to show the presence of the virus in the T cells. This was done with EBV in the B cells of patients with Burkitt's lymphoma and infectious mononucleosis. The use of molecular probes to detect the presence of known agents that cannot be passed to target cells is underway in a number of laboratories.

Summary

The Acquired Immune Deficiency Syndrome is most likely caused by a virus infection. I propose that an initial virus infection results in an immune deficiency that permits the development of Kaposi's sarcoma, which may be due to a viral infection (CMV), or the development of lymphomas, which may be due to a viral infection (EBV). The immune deficiency also permits the development of multiple opportunistic infections of various types including unusually severe, life-threatening virus infections due to known and perhaps undescribed viruses.

Some of the viruses causing symptomatic disease are candidates for the virus that causes the immunodeficiency. If this is so, there must be something different about strains of these known viruses (e.g., CMV, EBV, HBV, delta virus) from previous strains. To differentiate new strains from old or to find the new virus is clearly going to be difficult and require collaborative programs among clinicians, epidemiologists, and basic scientists who are willing to devote considerable time and cooperative effort in solving this most perplexing and alarming problem.

6

Bacterial and Mycotic Infections

Donald B. Louria, M.D.

Perhaps one of every three or four patients hospitalized with AIDS will develop or manifest at least one and often two or more of the bacterial, yeast, and fungal infections discussed in this paper. The candida infection ordinarily remains localized and is annoying but not lethal. On the other hand, the mycobacterial, cryptococcal, and nocardial infections are often lethal. Even though we possess potent antimicrobials against some of these infections, a certain percentage of severely immune-compromised patients will die of the infections despite adequate therapy. This percentage may well be the greater in AIDS patients. At present there is no predictably effective regimen for treatment of at least one of these superinfections.

Complications of the Acquired Immune Deficiency Syndrome can be divided into four categories; superficial yeast infections; systemic yeast infections; a farrago of higher bacterial and true fungal infections; and other bacterial infections.

Superficial Yeast Infections

These have supervened in more than 20 percent of AIDS cases reported to the Centers for Disease Control and are uniformly due to pathogenic species of candida (monilia). The site of infection is almost invariably the mouth and esophagus; surprisingly there are virtually no cases of systemic spread to involve deep-seated tissues such as kidneys or heart. Thus this form of candidiasis is much like that observed in:

- infants suffering from congenital immunodeficiency syndromes such as the DiGeorge's syndrome in which there is absence of the thymus;
- infants and children who have endocrine deficiencies including hypoadrenalism, hypoparathyroidism, and hypothyroidism;
- adults who have underlying thymoma; and
- young persons who have unexplained defects in delayed immune mechanisms manifested by failure to respond to a battery of skin test antigens that elicit a delayed response in 24–48 hours.

Unlike these other groups, the patients with the acquired immune deficiency syndrome develop nail involvement far less often and none has manifested the grotesque excrescences characteristic of monilial granuloma. In one case the candidal lesions were located in the axilla and groin.[1]

The mouth-esophageal candidiasis may precede any other superinfection, may occur concomitantly with other more serious infections, or may appear after the diagnosis of AIDS is well established.

The following two apposite cases illustrate these clinical presentations.

CASE 1

A thirty-year-old female drug addict and prostitute was admitted with a six-month history of weight loss, fever, lethargy, and apathy. She complained of sore throat and difficulty in swallowing. Physical examination and laboratory studies revealed a cachetic female with hair loss, fever, anemia, lymphopenia, and anergy. Intractable oral and esophageal candidiasis was found.

This occurred in 1980 before the AID syndrome had been fully recognized. We carried out a comprehensive work-up to explain the presence of the candida infection. Aside from anergy, no underlying defect was found that would account for the refractory monilial infection. Despite administration of oral nystatin, the oral-esophageal candidiasis persisted. She was subsequently rehospitalized because of shortness of breath and a diffuse pulmonary infiltrate that progressed inexorably. Although no autopsy was performed, we realized one year later that she had almost certainly suffered from AIDS and that the unexplained lethal pneumonia was probably due to *Pneumocystis carinii*.

CASE 2

A twenty-eight-year-old intravenous user of heroin and cocaine was hospitalized because of fever and bilateral patchy pulmonary infiltrates. A cardiac systolic murmur was present and a tentative diagnosis of staphylococcal tricuspid endocarditis was made. On admission, no pharyngeal abnormalities were present, but one day later he developed extensive oral candidiasis. This finding by itself completely changed the diagnostic assumptions. We were now sure he had AIDS and that his lung infiltrates were probably due to *Pneumocystis carinii*. Blood cultures showed no growth but the lung lesions expanded, necessitating open lung biopsy to establish a microbiological diagnosis. Many *Pneumocystis carinii* organisms were seen on histologic section. Despite vigorous therapy the lung infection fulminated and caused death. The oral-esophageal candidiasis had responded to oral administration of large amounts of nystatin.

Comment

The response to therapy is completely unpredictable.[2] In some cases the candida infection resolves after orally administered nonabsorbed anti-candida agents; in others the infection persists until intravenous amphotericin B or oral ketoconazole is administered; and in still others the infection resists all therapeutic attempts and either persists or relapses as soon as treatment is stopped. There are also cases in which the oral candidiasis seems to have resolved spontaneously.

Thus, in the patient with AIDS, monilia infections occur frequently, may be the first clinical evidence of the syndrome, and may be very helpful diagnostically. Certainly the presence of florid, unexplained mouth and esophageal candidiasis in a young person should mandate a careful epidemiologic and sexual exposure history as well as a search for immunologic abnormalities and other superinfections that characterize the AID syndrome. It is virtually inevitable that there will be reported cases in which the severe esophageal candidiasis results in esophageal perforation. It is also inevitable that systemic candida infection will occasionally be reported in this population. In one case presented at the Intercity Infectious Diseases Rounds by the Infectious Diseases group at St. Luke's–Roosevelt Hospital Center, disseminated candidiasis occurred late in the course of the patient's illness as a preterminal event after antibiotics and intravenous medications and fluids had been given via an indwelling vascular catheter. A similar case was reported by Fainstein et al.[3] The patient did not apparently have oral-esophageal candidiasis. Prior to evidence of disseminated candidiasis he was given multiple immunosuppressant anti-tumor agents as well as adrenal steroids and developed neutropenia, all these being risk factors for the supervention of disseminated candida infection. In a third case autopsy showed *Pneumocystis carinii* and cytomegalovirus infections as well as systemic candidiasis involving the lung and adrenal gland.[4] Cases of isolated lung and bladder candidiasis have also been reported.[5] If any patient (with or without AIDS) has superficial candidiasis, is treated with antibiotics, and has indwelling vascular catheters, systemic candidiasis is likely to occur.

Since clinical and experimental evidence strongly support the notion that the polymorphonuclear leukocyte is the most important host defense in systemic candida infection and since there is no evidence of a polymorph defect in the AID syndrome, these patients should have little proclivity to systemic candida infection. Their extraordinary deficiency in delayed-type immune mechanisms, on the other hand, should enhance their susceptibility to mucocutaneous candidiasis, a form of candida infection whose control is dependent on delayed type hypersensitivity. Two studies suggest, however, that there may not be such a strict dichotomy in defense mechanisms against mucocutaneous and systemic candidiasis. Diamond and Haudenschild have shown that monocytes damage hyphal forms of *Candida albicans*,[6] and we have found that experimental systemic candida infections can be augmented by blockage of late (presumable lymphocyte-mediated) candida tissue clearance.

Systemic Yeast Infections

This category includes only a single agent, *Cryptococcus neoformans* (or rarely other cryptococci). At the time of this symposium less than 100 cases of cryptococcal infection in AIDS patients have been reported to the Centers for Disease Control, but this undoubtedly represents substantial under-reporting. Like toxoplasmosis, the nature of cryptococcal infection is often inexplicably different in these patients. In part this may be a concatenation of two disparate phenomena—the presence of an extraordinarily compromised host (the AIDS patient) and a change in the yeast itself. In the pre-antimicrobial era the yeast *Cryptococcus neoformans*, a ubiquitous organism that grows particularly well in pigeon droppings, caused isolated meningitis in both normals and in those compromised by certain diseases, particularly lymphoma of the Hodgkin's type. In the last two decades extra-central nervous system cryptococcosis has been observed more frequently, involving particularly the lungs, bone, and genito-urinary system. At least half the patients with cryptococcal infection of these sites outside the nervous system have suffered from underlying disease, usually hematologic malignancies. The cryptococcal infection ordinarily surfaces during treatment—often with a combination of adrenal steroids and immunosuppressive agents—of the underlying disease. In recent years the yeast has been recovered from the peripheral blood in a substantial number of cases, whereas in the decades prior to 1970 detection of cryptococci in blood cultures was a rarity. This may be due to better isolation techniques by the various microbiology laboratories, or possibly there has been a change in the yeast itself. There is no direct evidence of a change in the cryptococcus that would permit its more ready isolation from blood cultures, but during this period microbiologic isolation techniques have improved. Furthermore, the pool of hosts who might develop cryptococcal fungemia has increased appreciably. The alternate possibility—that the yeast has increased in virulence or in its capacity to gain access to the bloodstream—has never been adequately tested in a well-standardized animal model.

The unusual aspects of cryptococcosis seen in AID syndrome patients are well illustrated by the following two cases.

CASE 3

A twenty-two-year-old male musician, who used marijuana but no other drugs and traveled widely throughout the United States, was hospitalized for weight loss, generalized myalgias, fever, and cough. His temperature was 103°F. by rectum and there was generalized non-tender lymphadenopathy. Fundoscopic examination showed multiple exudates and hemorrhages. Liver function studies were normal but subsequently showed a modest alkaline phosphatase elevation. Cerebrospinal fluid showed 100 cells, all lymphocytes, a glucose of 12 mg/dl and a protein of 70 mg/dl. Cultures of blood, bone marrow, urine, lymph node biopsy, and liver biopsy all showed *Cryptococcus neoformans*. No other disease was evident in either liver or lymph nodes. There were hordes of cryptococci in the tissues with either no host response or poorly formed granulomas. Cerebrospinal fluid antigen titer was 1:2048 and serum antigen titer was 1:16384.

He was married and fervently denied either intravenous drug use or homosexuality. He subsequently acknowledged a period of several months about a year prior to his illness of homosexual behavior of a relatively nonpromiscuous nature.

The cryptococcal infection responded surprisingly well to a combination of amphotericin B and 5 fluorocytosine, given over a three-month period. Cerebrospinal fluid antigen titer rose to 1:4096, then fell progressively to 1:16. He remained reasonably well for three months, then developed fulminating pneumonia thought to be due to *Pneumocystis carinii*. He died shortly after an open lung biopsy was performed. The biopsy showed no *Pneumocystis carinii* but massive infection with *Mycobacterium avium-intracellulare*. At autopsy there was no residual cryptococcal infection evident.

CASE 4

A thirty-year-old man who was a heavy drinker and possibly a homosexual was hospitalized for fever, chills, nausea, and dark urine. Sclerae were jaundiced and the liver was enlarged. He had marked and persistent lymphopenia. Two days after admission he developed lethargy, confusion, diarrhea, and a generalized maculo-papular, pustular, and vesicular rash. Lumbar puncture showed 76 red blood cells/mm^3, no white blood cells, a glucose of 10 mg/dl, and a protein of 40 mg/dl. Blood, urine, skin lesions, and spinal fluid showed *Cryptococcus neoformans* on culture; cerebrospinal fluid antigen titer was 1:4096. Toxoplasma titers were strongly positive (indirect fluorescent antibody IgM 1:512, IgG 1:256).

Despite therapy with amphotericin B and 5 fluorocytosine, he died.

Comment

Among the unusual aspects of these cases are the height of the antigen titer, the adenopathy due to *C. neoformans* invasion, and the ease of recovery of the organism from a great many sites including the bloodstream. The vesicular and pustular rash observed in the second case is extraordinary for cryptococcal infection. In one case, described by Mildvan et al.,[7] lethal cryptococcal respiratory infection occurred over forty-eight hours in an AIDS patient with extrapulmonary crypto-coccosis.

Among the reported cases[8] and a substantial number seen at various infectious disease rounds, there is no single clinical or thera-peutic response pattern. Some have had very high antigen titers (>1:1000); others have had much lower titers or even negative titers. Some patients have had the cryptococcus discovered at autopsy; others have died despite treatment, as in our second case; and still others responded well to appropriate therapy, as in our first case.

Because the cryptococcal infections tend to be widespread and the host is unable to contribute significantly to control of the yeast, dual therapy with amphotericin B and 5 fluorocytosine is, I believe, to be recommended for all cases. There is likely to be consensus about this recommendation for those with central nervous system involvement, but some may argue that, pending more data, amphotericin B alone is satisfactory for infection not involving the nervous system. Miconazole and ketoconazole, two anti-fungal and anti-yeast imidazoles, have at most a secondary role in treatment of AIDS patients suffering from cryptococcal superinfection.

Higher Bacterial and True Fungal Infections

Among the higher bacteria the most prevalent superinfecting organisms have been *Mycobacterium tuberculosis* and *Mycobacterium avium-intracellulare*, an organism that appears to be assuming increas-ing importance in other situations as well. This ubiquitous organism is in the Runyon group III category, is a non-chromogen, and is an amalgamation of two very closely related atypical mycobacteria, *Myco-bacterium avium* and *Mycobacterium intracellulare*. Lung, liver, spleen, lymph nodes, and bone marrow are the tissues most frequently involved.[9] Histologically the reaction to *M. avium-intracellulare* inva-sion is extraordinarily variable in AIDS patients: in some myriads of organisms are seen without significant tissue reaction, in others there are nonspecific tissue changes, in still others poorly formed granulomas are noted, and sometimes caseating or non-caseating granulomas are found. In some cases, as in our case 3, the *M. avium-intracellulare* is found only preterminally or at autopsy. Others have been treated with two to six anti-mycobacterial drugs including rifampin, isoniazid, ethambutol, ethionamide, streptomycin, capreomycin, cycloserine, and pyrazinamide, but the organisms tend to be highly resistant *in vitro* and almost invariably the infection persists, progresses, or relapses. Two new agents, ansamycin and clofazimine, are now undergoing trial. Ansamycin is a rifampicin derivative; if administered rifampin should be discontinued. Clofazimine is an anti-leprosy agent that appears reasonably effective *in vitro*.

Disseminated *M. avium-intracellulare* infections are usually fatal in non-AIDS cases, but there have been recoveries even when the organism isolated appears resistant *in vitro* to the agents used.[10] Of the approximately twenty cases thus far reported in AIDS patients, there is to my knowledge only one apparently successfully treated case—a patient whose remission coincided with ansamycin treatment.[11] I am aware of another patient who responded well clinically to anti-tuberculosis drugs but bone marrow examination continues to show occasional acid-fast organisms. In a third case *M. avium-intracellulare* was cultivated from a lung biopsy but there was no evidence it was causing disease.[12] Although the case fatality rate is over 90 percent it is important to emphasize that late diagnosis and the presence of other disseminated infections (including pneumocystosis and cytomegalovirus infection) or Kaposi's sarcoma contribute to the bleak prognosis once *M. avium-intracellulare* infection supervenes.

The following is a typical case.

CASE 5

A twenty-six-year-old Haitian man who had emigrated to the United States in 1978 was hospitalized for fever, weight loss, and oral thrush. Skin lesions were present on the buttocks and cultures of these ulcers showed herpes simplex. Because of abnormal liver function tests, a liver biopsy was performed. This showed poorly formed granulomas teeming with acid-fast bacilli; cultures showed *M. avium-intracellulare*. He was treated with isoniazid, rifampin, pyrazinamide, and ethambutol without response and subsequently died of an overwhelming nosocomially acquired bacterial pneumonia.

An increasing number of cases of *Mycobacterium tuberculosis* have also been reported. In one series of 10 AIDS cases arising in Haitian men, 6 had tuberculosis as one of their infections;[13] in another series, 9 of 20 patients had disseminated tuberculosis.[14] According to the Centers for Disease Control about 3 percent of AIDS cases have had concomitant or complicating tuberculosis; but the number is still small enough that it is not yet possible to relate these cases specifically to the underlying AID syndrome. Before this can be done we will need solid epidemiologic evidence on the prevalence of tuberculosis in a demographically similar population without AID syndrome. This is especially true for Haitians, whose incidence of tuberculosis is still substantial.[15] However, the human tubercle bacillus is handled by host delayed-immune mechanisms, and in view of the profound sundering of the effectiveness of that defense system in AIDS patients, it seems logical that tuberculosis would supervene in these patients. Whether their response to anti-tuberculosis medications will be diminished is not yet known.

A few cases of other mycobacterial and *Nocardia asteroides* infections have also been reported. Since the few experimental and the more extensive clinical data available suggest that *Nocardia asteroides* invasion is handled by the lymphocyte-macrophage system,[16] such infections would be expected. However, studies by Felice and colleagues[17] showing that neither human neutrophils nor human monocytes kill *N. asteroides* emphasize that our knowledge of defense mechanisms against *N. asteroides* is still rudimentary.

The following is a case observed recently by our group.

CASE 6

A thirty-four-year-old female drug addict was admitted in June 1982 with a history of low-grade fever, abnormal liver function studies, and bilateral infiltrates in the chest. The liver was enlarged and tender, and florid oral candidiasis was present. She was anergic and lymphopenic. A liver biopsy demonstrated alcoholic hepatitis. Sputum smears and cultures showed normal flora and no evidence of tuberculosis.

Bronchoscopy with transbronchial biopsy showed *Pneumocystis carinii*, and she was treated for three weeks with trimethoprim-sulfamethoxazole. This resulted in significant improvement in the pulmonary lesions. She was also given ketoconazole, 200 mg daily by mouth, and this effected striking improvement in the oral thrush. She was subsequently discharged on a regimen of vitamin supplementation and a high protein diet.

Four weeks after discharge she noted fever and headache and then developed blurring of vision bilaterally. These symptoms increased progressively, necessitating hospitalization. Physical examination on admission showed papilledema indicative of increased intracranial pressure but there were no focal neurological signs. A computerized tomographic study revealed a clover-shaped brain abscess. Because the etiology of the brain lesion was unclear, brain biopsy was done. Cultures of the abscess material showed both *Salmonella enteriditis* and *Nocardia asteroides*. Shortly after the brain biopsy, she died.

Comment

This is an extraordinary case. Both organisms recovered from the brain abscess are handled by delayed immune mechanisms and her delayed-type immunity had been vitiated by the AID syndrome. She manifested two of the most frequently observed infectious complications, pulmonary pneumocystosis and oral thrush, as well as an unusual superinfection due to a species of nocardia and a bacterial infection due to a group of organisms, the salmonellae, being reported with increasing frequency. The site of the salmonella infection is very unusual indeed. To our knowledge this is the first report in this population of a salmonella brain abscess and the first report in any patient population of a combined nocardial-salmonella brain abscess.

The treatment of choice for nocardial infection is now trimethoprim-sulfamethoxazole or a sulfonamide alone. There is great variability in sensitivity of individual nocardia strains to anti-microbials and it is important that *in vitro* susceptibility tests be carried out. There are too few cases in AID syndrome patients to make a judgment about differential response to therapy compared to non-AIDS patients.

In AID syndrome patients only a small number of superinfections have been reported that are caused by the true fungi, *Histoplasma capsulatum*, *Coccidioides immitis*, and *Blastomyces dermatitidis*. Since the available evidence suggests the importance of delayed immunity in at least histoplasmosis and coccidioidomycosis, their supervention would be readily understood. The paucity of cases is analogous to the situation in hematologic malignancy of the Hodgkin's lymphoma type, in which there is a monolithic defect in delayed-type hypersensitivity but in which superinfections with these three fungi occur only infrequently and then usually after the disease-induced host defect is augmented by anti-tumor therapy.[18]

A few cases of aspergillus superinfection have been described. This is surprising since the primary host defense against aspergilli is thought to be the polymorphonuclear leukocyte. However, recent studies have shown the efficacy of monocytes in damaging or killing aspergillus hyphae[19] and it may well be that an optimal host response requires the activity of both the polymorphonuclear leukocyte and the monocyte-macrophage system. Still, it is a bit surprising that aspergilli would be the offending superinfection pathogens in these patients, and as with candidiasis, this may be a late manifestation after a variety of medications have been given.

Other Bacterial Infections

These patients may develop pneumonias due to a variety of bacteria, but there are no persuasive data to relate these pneumonias to increased susceptibility induced by the AID syndrome. In most instances the pneumonias occur late in the course during hospitalization after massive weight loss and treatment for other infections or Kaposi's sarcoma. The only two bacteria that appear to be related to the AID syndrome are salmonella and shigella. The latter is found frequently in homosexual men who do not have evidence of the AID syndrome and the data do not permit a conclusion about a possible increase once the AID syndrome occurs. Intestinal and/or systemic salmonella infections have been reported to the Centers for Disease Control in only a small number of instances but there are obvious problems of under-reporting. Although salmonella infections have been reported only infrequently in adults, four of eight children acquiring the disease in the first year of life have had salmonella infection, a disturbingly high percentage.[20] In three cases the salmonella invaded the bloodstream, whereas in the fourth case repeated intestinal infection occurred.

The following is a case observed by my colleague Dr. Flor Tecson and her associates at the Veterans Administration Hospital in East Orange, New Jersey.

Case 7

A thirty-five-year-old bisexual man developed multiple skin lesions found on biopsy to be Kaposi's sarcoma. He was hospitalized because of weight loss and diarrhea. In the past stool cultures had shown no pathogens. Thrush was evident on examination of the oral cavity. On admission he was febrile to 102.8°F. by rectum and over the next forty-eight hours his apparent infection fulminated. A diagnosis of gram negative sepsis was made and mezlocillin and tobramycin were given. On advice of the infectious diseases consultants ampicillin and trimethoprim-sulfamethoxazole were added, but he died three hours later. *Salmonella enteriditis* was recovered from both blood and stool cultures.

Comment

I am absolutely certain on the basis of our own observations that salmonella infections will be reported with increasing frequency. As with oral candidiasis, the presence of salmonella bacteremia or recurrent gastrointestinal salmonellosis in a child of less than one year of age or in any young adult without obvious reasons (such as travel to underdeveloped areas) should compel the physician to give careful consideration to the possible presence of AID syndrome. The few data now available suggest that these patients respond adequately to antibiotic therapy (e.g., ampicillin, chloramphenicol, trimethoprim-sulfamethoxazole). Progressive, lethal salmonellosis despite appropriate therapy has not yet, to my knowledge, been reported, but recurrent salmonellosis has, suggesting that the AIDS host defects may promote persistence of the salmonella organisms. In the case described above death occurred so soon after anti-salmonella therapy was given and the disease was so fulminating and had progressed so far before such treatment was initiated that this death cannot be designated an antimicrobial failure. Recently an extraordinary case of salmonella endocarditis was reported in a twenty-four-year-old Haitian man.[21] I know of only one instance of superinfection with *Listeria monocytogenes;* reports of infection with this organism should increase since delayed immune mechanisms are paramount in defense against *L. monocytogenes*.

Some Final Thoughts

These superinfections force AIDS patients to undergo prolonged hospitalization and contribute further to the weight loss patterns that often give them the appearance of prisoners in concentration camps.

This nutritional dwindling in a hospital milieu increases their susceptibility to quiescent infections they have already acquired outside the hospital, to infections with their own indigenous flora, and to hospital-based organisms. Their stay in the hospital also increases the likelihood that some indigenous or exogenous pathogens will acquire antibiotic resistance factors. I would be willing to predict that not only will salmonella infections be reported with increasing frequency but also that there will be cases in which, during an acute bacteremia episode or during recurrences, initially susceptible salmonellae will become broadly antimicrobial-resistant and then may even cause intrahospital epidemics, a contretemps we experienced several years ago in a non-AIDS patient.[22]

One possibility in treatment of cryptococcal, mycobacterial, nocardial, and candida infections is the administration of transfer factor. There is at present no evidence that transfer factor will alter the devastating underlying defect, but such treatment might be beneficial for two reasons.

1. It may produce a fugacious increase in specific resistance that would allow the antimicrobials to be more effective.
2. There is evidence in experimental mouse candidiasis that transfer factor (leukocyte dialysate) exerts a small but measurable beneficial effect that is nonspecific.[23] This might be very helpful in severely ill persons.

Surely this therapeutic modality is worth a try if the infection is recusant in antibiotic-response or recurrent. This would particularly apply to systemic *Mycobacterium avium-intracellulare* infections and to oral-esophageal candidiasis. Such treatment has been given in at least three cases of *M. avium-intracellulare* infection and may have helped in one instance.[24]

Presumably there is nothing we can do to prevent these superinfections once the immunologic deficits of the syndrome have become established. However, we all have been impressed with the profound and often persistent weight loss in these patients. Indeed, if during or after therapy for a given superinfection, these patients continue to lose weight, we have informed the relatives that recurrent infection and death is virtually inevitable. We clearly do not know enough about specific nutritional deficits, especially relating to vitamins and trace metals. It would seem likely that the weight loss is associated with profound specific nutrient decrements that may vitiate delayed immune mechanism further. For example, it is well known that protein-calorie malnutrition, zinc deficits, and pyridoxine deficiency may be associated with reversible decrements in delayed immune mechanisms.[25] It would seem advisable to carefully study the nutritional status of AIDS patients prior to and during periods of weight loss. Nutritional status has been assessed reasonably carefully in one study[26] and zinc levels have been found to be normal in nine cases,[27] but many more data are needed, including determinations of other trace metals and circulating vitamin concentrations. My colleague, Dr. Rajendra Kapila, is at present conducting such a study. It might well be that some of the profound host defects might relate to specific nutritional deficiencies and that their correction might either prevent certain infectious complications or increase the effectiveness of antimicrobial therapy.

Finally, it seems to me we must be both rigid and cautious in our case definitions. There is a growing tendency to include in the AIDS rubric any person who has unexplained *Pneumocystis carinii* infection or particular combinations of infections. It would be tempting, for example, to try to force, even without adequate evidence, the case described by Gentry and associates of combined central nervous system infection with *Cryptococcus neoformans* and *Mycobacterium avium-intracellulare*[28] into the AIDS category. Once an infection has occurred it is not even clear that helper/suppressor cell ratio determinations will aid appreciably in case definition. This concern applies to our case 4, who is being classified by us as a probable AIDS case because of the nature of the cryptococcal infection and the persuasive serologic evidence of an active toxoplasma infection. Until we have better markers for the disease (perhaps viral infection markers) we will have to be careful that we do not become too inclusive in our case ascertainment, for this might confound our search for etiologic clues and would certainly add to the growing apprehension about a disease that at least in its clinically evident form carries a high case-fatality rate and whose frequency appears to be increasing at an alarming rate.

7

Parasitic Infections

Kevin M. Cahill, M.D.

More AIDS patients die from parasitic infections than from any other cause. That is a striking revelation, particularly in a nation that has for generations dismissed parasitic diseases as interesting but exotic problems of peasants in the poor, developing lands of the world. The majority of American medical schools offer no instruction in clinical parasitology. Few physicians in the United States have had any experience in the diagnosis and management of these ailments. Yet the diseases that were once so easily—if erroneously—relegated to "tropical" medicine are now a critical part of the puzzle in the present AIDS epidemic.

Pneumocystis carinii Pneumonia (PCP)

The most common cause of death in AIDS is a pulmonary parasite, *Pneumocystis carinii*. It is an unusual organism with a fascinating history. First described in 1909 by Chagas, whose name rests securely in the history of medicine as the discoverer of South American trypanosomiasis, the parasite was not even identified as a human pathogen till the late 1930s. Then, during World War II, localized outbreaks of PCP occurred in malnourished children, and many workers, myself included, have since had experience with this highly fatal infection during epidemics and famine in refugee camps. In the United States the first adult case was observed only in 1954, and until the present AIDS epidemic virtually all PCP patients were immune-compromised persons receiving cancer chemotherapy or organ transplants.

While serologic studies indicate that many people are exposed to pneumocystis, there have been no documented clinical cases of PCP in an adult with an intact immune protective system. This observation is of great comfort to physicians, nurses, and other health workers who must currently care for AIDS victims.

Clinical Manifestations

Most AIDS patients have been ill for some time when they give evidence of PCP. Weight loss, fever, drenching night sweats, diarrhea, and unexplained lymph node enlargement usually precede the patient's pulmonary complaints. The onset of PCP is often insidious, with only minor symptoms of a dry, nonproductive cough. The infection is rarely detected at this early stage because the level of clinical awareness is low, the complaints are so vague and nonspecific, and, as we shall see, the diagnosis is both technically difficult and the picture complicated by other invasive pathogens.

In about 25 percent of the AIDS patients with PCP that I have examined, the onset is more fulminant, with marked shortness of breath, particularly on exertion. Patients try to compensate by rapid shallow breathing, but are frequently cyanotic. Diffuse moist rales and rhonchi can be heard through the stethoscope, and retraction of the ribs may be seen.

Diagnosis

Since AIDS victims are peculiarly susceptible to cytomegalic virus, tuberculosis, and other atypical mycobacterial organisms, and to a wide range of bacterial lung infections, it is obviously essential to identify *Pneumocystis carinii* organisms before concluding that a patient with pulmonary signs and symptoms has PCP. It is extremely unusual to detect the parasites by concentrated sputum analysis, and medicine currently offers no effective methods for either culturing pneumocystis in the laboratory or isolating them by animal inoculation. Thus, one is forced to obtain material directly from the lung; the flexible bronchoscope is the preferred tool to accomplish this.

Bronchoscopy is an invasive procedure and should be done only by trained pulmonary specialists in a hospital setting. The illuminated tube permits direct visualization of the bronchial tree, and brushings from the wall and transbronchial biopsies of the lung provide the needed specimens for analysis. Impression smears stained with silver methanamine permit immediate examination and offer the best chance to identify the typical small (4–6 μm) cysts singly or in clusters, with up to eight intracellular meozoites. Staining does not, however, permit the pathologist to distinguish between live and killed cysts. This is a critical problem since the viability of pneumocystis cannot currently be determined by culture methods, and the clinician is often faced with the unhappy dilemma of having to decide whether to administer or withhold therapy purely on morphologic grounds. Quantitative parasite counts on impression smears can offer a rough guideline to the severity of PCP, but particularly in sequential bronchoscopies done on a single patient during therapy, they have proved a disappointing parameter.

Histologic specimens in AIDS patients are rarely positive if the impression smears are negative. This finding seems to be at variance with the common experience in PCP patients receiving cancer chemotherapy and in the immune-compromised organ transplant group. Nevertheless, paraffin-fixed specimens do provide important information regarding the extent of damage and, during therapy, of progress or lack thereof. In severe cases of PCP in our AIDS group, almost all alveoli are filled with masses of parasitic cysts and an eosinophilic proteinaceous material producing a pattern that has been described as a "tightly woven honeycomb." This pathology clearly explains the difficulties PCP patients have exchanging oxygen and carbon dioxide.

Blood gas determinations are usually deranged in PCP, with severe hypoxemia often seen even in the absence of clinical cyanosis. Following serial anterial oxygen levels offers a reasonable prognostic monitor in measuring response to therapy. None of the other routine laboratory blood studies are of particular value in diagnosis.

Chest X rays are the obvious choice for the physician wishing to visually assess and follow a patient with PCP. There are serious limitations, however, for there is frequently a lag period of at least several days between a deteriorating clinical picture in PCP and demonstrable X-ray changes. Chest X rays may, in fact, appear perfectly normal in PCP when a simultaneous gallium scan indicates active pulmonary pathology and a lung biopsy confirms pneumocystis infection. This normal X ray/severe clinical disease pattern has been seen in 50 percent of my recent PCP cases.

Serial X-ray studies will show the progression in PCP from a diffuse ground-glass pattern characteristic of interstitial lung damage to a later picture of focal consolidation with marked hilar adenopathy. Since concomitant lung infections with various viral and bacterial agents are common, it is sometimes difficult to attribute all the X-ray changes noted to PCP. Both the gallium scan and X ray can help the broncho-scopist to select a likely area for biopsy, but they are not a substitute basis for accurate diagnosis; one must identify *Pneumocystis carinii* organisms to make a diagnosis of PCP.

Extrapulmonary pneumocystis invasion of many organs has been reported. In the AIDS patients, involvement of the eye has been proved recently, and PCP may be responsible for the cotton-wool exudate seen in the fundi of many AIDS victims. Although various viruses can produce the same retinal changes, the correlation of visual defects with PCP in AIDS is striking. As with so many other aspects of the present epidemic, this observation does not offer an answer, but merely the beginning of a series of questions.

Therapy

Specific chemotherapy for PCP is available and highly effective, but the underlying immunologic defect in AIDS patients makes imme-diate treatment failure common and recurrence of pneumonia within a year unfortunately frequent. Also, AIDS patients with pneumocystis infection appear to require longer courses and higher doses of medica-tion than those with PCP complicating cancer chemotherapy or organ transplantation. Two drugs are used, alone or in combination, in treating PCP.

Bactrim (trimethoprim-sulfamethoxazole) is usually employed as the first line of therapy. A total daily dosage of 20 mg/kg trimethoprim and 100 mg/kg of sulfamethoxazole can be administered either orally or intravenously, depending on the severity of the illness. The standard course of fourteen days often proves inadequate and one must then either prolong the course or switch to a pentamidine regimen.

My own bias is toward pentamidine, but that reflects a previous personal experience with this compound in treating African trypanosomiasis and the underlying fear that I harbor for the suppressive side effects of Bactrim in already compromised patients. Most AIDS patients enter therapy with a low white blood cell count and Bactrim, in my experience, almost always produces an even more severe leukopenia, leaving the patient very vulnerable to all other infections. It is for this same reason that I do not employ Bactrim "prophylaxis" after

FIGURE 1

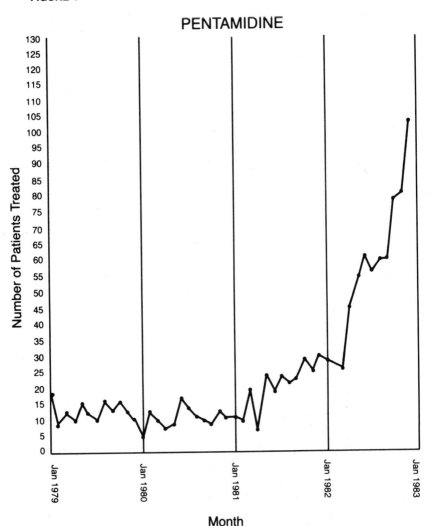

treating PCP in the AIDS group. The speculative benefit does not, to me, seem worth the risk.

Pentamidine is not without its problems, and my personal preference for this drug is combined with a healthy respect for the adverse reactions it can cause. Once again the standard fourteen-day course of intramuscular injections of 4 mg/kg must often be extended. Several of my patients have required more than twice that amount over at least double the duration before clinical and histologic clearing is observed. Almost 50 percent of patients receiving an extended course of pentamidine will develop deterioration of kidney function, but this is usually transient and will respond to careful fluid management and adequate hydration. Painful abscesses at the infection sites can occur and temporary hypotension may be a problem. Clinical medicine often offers a choice between unpleasant options and, at least in my experience, pentamidine provides a better cure rate with fewer life-threatening side effects than the more easily administered Bactrim. One of the minor obstacles facing the clinician desiring to use pentamidine is the fact that it is not generally available for sale in the United States. It can be obtained free by requesting it from the Centers for Disease Control (CDC). Despite that difficulty, many physicians treating PCP in AIDS are becoming new devotees of an old compound (Figure 1).

Until many more PCP patients in the AIDS group are treated with various regimens, the choice of a specific drug and the length of treatment will remain more in the realm of the art rather than the science of medicine.

Toxoplasmosis

Another parasitic complication of AIDS, far less frequent than PCP but more often fatal, is toxoplasmosis. As with pneumocystis, *Toxoplasma gondii* is an opportunistic parasite that is presumed to have been present in many patients for long periods as a latent, asymptomatic infection that is then activated as the individual's immunity is compromised. Its appearance as part of the AIDS pattern is, therefore, not surprising. Even that heightened awareness, however, has not eased the clinician's difficulties in diagnosis or in deciding when and for how long to treat.

Toxoplasmosis in AIDS has been recognized largely as a catastrophic complication. Classic lymph node and ocular changes of adult-acquired toxoplasmosis have not been reported in AIDS victims. Rather, the disease seems to start at the terminal end of the spectrum.

As Magendie once described cholera—"a disease that begins where others end, with death"—so too is the fulminance with which toxoplasmosis presents in AIDS. The physician is frequently faced with signs of diffuse encephalopathy, meningoencephalitis, or a brain abscess in a rapidly deteriorating patient.

At this point in the current AIDS epidemic, the CDC is aware of some fifty cases of central nervous system (CNS) toxoplasmosis. Since the majority have been diagnosed at the autopsy table—a time and location for detection not to be commended—one can only speculate on the real incidence. Remington and his co-workers in California have recently collected twelve new cases (personal communication), and one can predict a steady increase as diagnostic techniques improve.

Diagnosis

The critical—indeed, indispensable—requirements for detection of toxoplasmosis in an AIDS patient are the awareness of the possibility and the willingness to aggressively pursue the suspicion. Standard serologic studies may not resolve the diagnostic dilemma. Most AIDS patients with toxoplasmosis will have elevated IfA/IgG levels but at a range far lower than expected even in other immune-compromised patients such as the cancer chemotherapy and organ transplant groups. Several AIDS patients with fatal toxoplasma brain abscesses have had negative or inconsequential toxoplasma titers. In the CDC study, the majority of AIDS patients who died from cerebral toxoplasmosis had not been serologically studied while alive. The first requirement, again, is to think of the possibility and not be dissuaded if the standard test criteria are not immediately satisfied.

Other relatively simple diagnostic tests have also proved disappointing. Despite the prevalence of enlarged lymph nodes in the AIDS population, Ioachim did not demonstrate the classic morphologic changes expected with toxoplasma lymphadenitis in a single case in a large series (personal communication). Examination of the spinal fluid in CNS toxoplasmosis usually shows an increase in protein and lymphocytes and, very rarely, even a toxoplasma organism. The CT scan can be very helpful in confirming the size, location, and, sometimes, the type of a destructive brain lesion. It also guides the search for a specific cause. Brain biopsy has become a necessary diagnostic tool in assessing an AIDS patient with CNS changes. One obviously approaches brain biopsy—or cardiac biopsy for the patient with sudden onset of acute heart failure—with great reluctance. Nevertheless, this technique has, in experienced hands, proved invaluable in confirming the presence of toxoplasma cysts. Armstrong and his colleagues have, in fact, followed a number of AIDS patients who have had repeated brain biopsies without serious complications. In most cases, however, the problem that faces a physician caring for AIDS patients is the rapid deterioration of an individual without a provable CNS diagnosis. Empiric therapy should be begun.

Therapy

If a seriously ill AIDS patient is suspected of having cerebral or cardiac toxoplasmosis, one should treat with sulfadiazine (4 gms per day) and pyrimethamine (a loading dose of 75 mg/kg for three days, followed by 25 mg/kg). The standard approach is to maintain therapy for three to four weeks, but whether this is sufficient for AIDS patients is questionable. These drugs do not destroy encysted *T. gondii* and complete cure is, therefore, never realized. Repetitive courses of treatment are the rule and, if possible, it may prove desirable to maintain AIDS patients who have had CNS toxoplasmosis on a sulfadiazine-pyrimethamine regimen for life. The limiting factor is the bone marrow–depressive side effect of the drug. This can be minimized by adding folinic acid.

Amebiasis and Giardiasis

Diarrhea, abdominal bloating, and excess intestinal gas are common complaints in New York's gay community. For at least a decade, physicians serving this group of patients have been aware of a high incidence of infection with *Entameba histolytica* (the parasite causing amebiasis) and *Giardia lamblia* (the etiologic agent of giardiasis). There have been numerous articles published on the "gay bowel syndrome," and the island of Manhattan has become well known as a focus for "tropical" infections. The vast majority of AIDS patients that I see in consultation have had previous diarrhea due to either or both of these amebic and giardia organisms. All AIDS patients should be examined for intestinal parasites.

Diagnosis

The value of a fecal analysis for ova and parasites depends on both the quality of the specimen and the talents—or incompetency—of the technologist. Stool specimens tend to be unpopular items in most laboratories, and are often assigned to the least experienced technician. Since the use of preserved stool specimens (using MIF or PVA) is uncommon, the clinician becomes unusually dependent on the transient observations of a technician. Whereas an X ray, cardiogram, and most other laboratory studies offer a permanent record that permits reevaluation or reinterpretation by a skeptical clinician, a stool analysis almost uniquely represents an act of faith in a particular laboratory. The confidence can be tragically misplaced. I have known certain laboratories to diagnose ameba in virtually every specimen, and "epidemics" of amebiasis or giardiasis can literally be traced to specific individuals and laboratories. Much of this overdiagnosis is due to inadequate training; undigested food particles, normal intestinal protozoa, and various bits of fecal debris are interpreted by the neophyte as pathogens and lead to dangerous courses of therapy. It is important for the physician to know the qualifications of his parasitologist; even more important, the good physician will learn to personally look down the microscope and challenge both negative and positive reports when they do not correlate with his clinical impression.

Furthermore, if a patient complained of a sore throat, the physician would not merely look at material expectorated; he would open the mouth and swab the throat to prepare a direct smear for analysis. So too should be the concerned physician's approach in amebiasis. Inserting a disposable proctoscope allows a view of the bowel wall and permits the doctor to scrape suspicious material directly from an inflamed area. A stool specimen is only a vehicle passing by; amebic organisms do not live in fecal material, they live in the bowel wall.

There are several other facets of fecal analysis that deserve attention. An unusual number of fat globules, for example, should heighten suspicion of upper intestinal malabsorption. They are often seen in patients with giardiasis. Charcot-Leyden crystals and ingested blood cells in trophozoites are good indicators of active amebiasis and should stimulate a continued search for the parasite. If organisms are not seen on direct saline smears, I normally use an ethyl acetate concentration method. Simultaneous cultivating for bacterial pathogens should always be done. Finally, a wide range of "interfering substances" can alter the accuracy of a stool study for parasites, and it is important to obtain specimens before any of these drugs or procedures are used (Table 1).

Amebic serology is not terribly helpful as a diagnostic aid in clinical interpretation of diarrhea in AIDS patients. Most patients with acute

Table 1
Interfering Treatments

Antidiarrheal preparations	Sulfonamides
Bismuth	Antibiotics
Clay	Antacids
Laxatives	X-ray procedures
Oils	Barium sulfate
Magnesium hydroxide	Enemas

intestinal amebiasis will have a negative result in any case. Even those with chronic disease may have a negative reaction due to the AIDS victim's inability to mount an adequate immunologic response.

X-ray studies can be helpful in diagnosing both amebiasis and giardiasis. The ragged ulcerations, narrowed cecum, and flattened villi patterns have been extensively described, and liver scans can be very helpful in assessing hepatomegaly when an amebic abscess becomes a serious part of a differential diagnosis.

Therapy

There are a number of excellent amebicidal drugs available. The cocktail-circuit conviction that one can never be cured of amebiasis is false. My current treatment of choice in New York is a combination of Humatin (paromomycin) and tetracycline for ten days. It is important to reexamine the patient at the end of therapy and, if still positive, to either prolong the course of therapy or switch to an alternative compound. Flagyl (metronidazole) is associated, in my experience, with far more adverse side effects and more frequent resistance. Carbasone and furamide are well-studied options. I do not use diiodoquin. There is no merit in employing all these drugs together or in sequence, a perverse practice recommended too often to patients in the gay community by doctors who apparently believe that a shotgun—or nuclear-bomb—approach must be better than a specific agent.

For giardiasis there are two drugs available, atabrine (quinacrine hydrochloride) or Flagyl. Both offer cure rates in the 85 to 90 percent range with a single course of therapy.

Cure as defined by the clinician consists of eradicating the harmful parasite. The patient, understandably, defines "cure" as the cessation of diarrhea, flatulence, or abdominal bloating. Since symptoms are due to damage to the patient's bowel wall, and since it may take two to three months for an ulcerated or destroyed bowel wall to return to normal, it is important to explain this "lag time" to the patient. Adherence to a bland diet and use of moderate antispasmodics are essential ingredients to ultimate but inevitable improvement.

Finally, it should be noted that reinfection is always possible with reexposure, especially in the sexually active.

Cryptosporidiasis

A new parasitic problem in AIDS patients is invasion by a coccidial protozoan that until less than a decade ago was recognized solely in turkeys, snakes, calves, lambs, and various rodents. Fulminant diarrhea has now been reported in many immune-compromised patients, and an almost choleralike syndrome with a daily loss of almost *twenty liters* of diarrheal fluid was seen in one AIDS victim for whom I consulted. However, most AIDS patients with cryptosporidia will present with minimal to moderate diarrhea with soft, mushy stools. In the few healthy persons who have accidentally acquired cryptosporidiasis from contact with infected animals, symptoms—and the cryptosporidia in stool specimens—vanished within two weeks without any specific therapy. In contrast, I have now followed over a dozen AIDS patients for more than six months with cryptosporidia constantly present in their feces; during that time they have ranged from being asymptomatic to suffering moderate abdominal cramping associated with five to ten watery bowel movements per day. I cannot correlate their intestinal remissions or exacerbations with diet or any other factor.

Diagnosis

Stool specimens submitted for analysis for cryptosporidia should be clearly labeled as such, specifically prepared with Sheather's sugar flotation method and Gremsa stain, and examined with phase contrast rather than bright-field microscopy. Isolation by inoculation into mice and rats can be done, but this is not practical in a general hospital laboratory. Biopsies of both the small and large intestine via endoscopy is also a useful method of demonstrating the parasite.

Therapy

There is no known effective treatment for human intestinal crypto-sporidiasis. Various drugs, including oral pentamidine, Flagyl, various antibiotics and antimalarials, have been tried, but no one has studied a sufficient number of cases to demonstrate efficacy. Supportive therapy and fluid replacement remain the basis for current clinical management.

8

Kaposi's Sarcoma

Bijan Safai, M.D.

In March of 1981 we came across a few cases of Kaposi's sarcoma in men who were much younger than expected for classical KS, all of whom were homosexuals. In addition, review of our autopsy reports indicated the occurrence of several such cases in 1979 and 1980 as well. At the same time, we were seeing cases of severe and fatal opportunistic infections (such as *Pneumocystis carinii* pneumonia, herpes simplex virus infections, and toxoplasmosis) in some young homosexual men who had no prior history of debilitating diseases and who were not being treated with immunosuppressive agents. The occurrence of KS at such a young age and the presence of fatal opportunistic infections in individuals who had no previous history of cancer or immunodeficiency was quite a striking and unusual experience for us. What was common to both groups was the fact that the patients were all homosexual men. Focusing on the sexual preference of these cases, it soon became clear that we had already seen several instances of homosexual men who presented with generalized lymphadenopathy of unknown nature and etiology, most of whom gave a history of lack of energy, loss of weight, malaise, and fatigue. Simultaneously at New York Hospital–Cornell University Medical College, cases of opportunistic infections, especially *Pneumocystis carinii* pneumonia (PCP), were being seen, while KS cases at New York University Medical

College and in San Francisco and cases of PCP in Los Angeles were being recorded. These observations resulted in two reports from the CDC in mid-1981 describing the outbreak of *Pneumocystis carinii* pneumonia and Kaposi's sarcoma in homosexual men. The epidemic nature of the outbreak was recognized when a steady increase in the number of cases was observed by us and others, and cases began to appear outside the metropolitan areas of New York and California. The number of cases increased from 41 in July of 1981 to 231 in February of 1982 and then to 340 in May of 1982 and reached over 1,000 cases by the end of that year. It became clear that what we observed initially was actually the tip of the iceberg (Figure 1), and that we are faced with a major epidemic of highly fatal disorders whose etiology is not as yet known. Table 1 shows the number of patients seen at Memorial Sloan-Kettering Cancer Center. In addition, a large and as yet untallied number of patients with generalized lymphadenopathy are being observed.

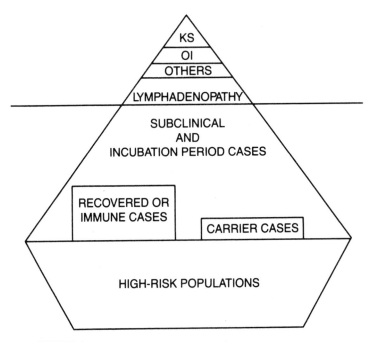

FIGURE 1
SPECTRUM OF DISORDERS SEEN IN EPIDEMIC OF AIDS

Table 1
Patients with AIDS Seen at MSKCC Since Beginning of the Epidemic

Date	KS	OI	LA
1978	—	1	—
1979	2	—	—
1980	2	—	1
Jan.–Feb. 81	—	—	—
Mar.–Apr. 81	1	—	—
May–Jun. 81	2	—	—
Jul.–Aug. 81	3	1	2
Sep.–Oct. 81	4	2	3
Nov.–Dec. 81	4	3	4
Jan.–Feb. 82	5	3	5
Mar.–Apr. 82	4	2	16
May–Jun. 82	4	3	13
Jul.–Aug. 82	9	6	12
Sep.–Oct. 82	12	3	13
Nov.–Dec. 82	12	5	7
Jan.–Feb. 83	12	3	11
Total	76	35	88

KS: Kaposi's sarcoma
OI: Opportunistic infections
LA: Generalized lymphadenopathy

History

Moriz Kaposi first described this condition as "idiopathic multiple pigmented sarcoma of the skin" in 1872. The disease was later named "Kaposi's sarcoma" at the suggestion of Koebner. Dr. Kaposi, however, called the disease "sarcoma idiopathicum multiplex hemorrhagicum," a name he believed more accurately described the condition and the source of pigment in the lesions.

Moriz Kaposi was born Moritz Kohn on October 23, 1837, in the regional trade center of Kaposvar on the river Kapos in southern Hungary. He graduated from Vienna University as doctor of medicine in 1861, doctor of surgery in 1862, and master of obstetrics in 1865. He became associate professor in 1866 and later a professor of dermatology in 1875. Dr. Kaposi became the Chairman of the Department of Dermatology, replacing Dr. Ferdinand Hebra, his father-in-law.

Dr. Kaposi described a slowly progressive disease in which violaceous nodules appear on the skin of the lower extremities. He reported the disease as a rare cutaneous disorder of adult men. He noted that the disease was not only multifocal on the skin but could involve the viscera and was frequently fatal. The three men he described in his initial report died within three years of diagnosis. The entity was then recognized in many countries. The first African case was reported in 1914 by Hallenberger, and later Smith and Elmes reported ten other cases of Kaposi's sarcoma. Other large series were also reported from Africa, following which the International Union Against Cancer held their meeting in Uganda in 1961 and concluded that 9 percent of all cancers in Uganda are Kaposi's sarcoma.

In the past two decades Kaposi's sarcoma has been observed with increasing incidence among renal transplant recipients and patients with immunologic disorders receiving immunosuppressive therapy. An increased occurrence of Kaposi's sarcoma has been recently recognized among young homosexual men in New York and California. Kaposi's sarcoma in this new population is part of the epidemic of Acquired Immune Deficiency Syndrome.

Incidence and Geographic Distribution

KS is a rare tumor except in certain endemic areas. It is estimated that KS is 200 times more frequent in Africa than in the United States. In the United States the incidence of classic KS is well below 1 percent of all cancers. Reynolds et al., in reviewing a thirty-eight-year experience at the Mayo Clinic, reported only 70 cases or 0.06 percent of tumors diagnosed at that center. Oettle and Dorn and Cutler have reported an even lower incidence of 0.02 per 100,000 in the United States, where it is mostly seen in persons of European descent. It is rare in American blacks and in those areas of West Africa where their ancestors originated.

KS has a cluster distribution and usually occurs in endemic areas. In Africa, KS is seen in Zaire, Kenya, and Tanzania, which are predominantly the hill and open savannah bush country, and native blacks are far more frequently affected than non-blacks. The geographic distribution of KS among the native population of equatorial Africa is similar to that of African Burkitt's lymphoma, a malignancy associated with Epstein-Barr virus. The high incidence of KS also parallels endemic malaria, which may facilitate a viral infection. In Europe, cases are mostly seen in Eastern Europe and Italy, or in individuals of Jewish extraction. In North America, the majority of patients with classical KS have ancestry going back to Eastern Europe or Italy.

Other cases have been also reported from Western Europe, Armenia, India, China, and Japan, but distinctly not as frequently as in endemic regions. KS has been reported in two persons with pure Eskimo heritage. In the series of ninety classical cases reported from Memorial Sloan-Kettering, most cases have been Italian or elderly Jewish men.

In the current epidemic of AIDS, KS cases have been seen more often among homosexual men than intravenous drug abusers. KS has not been so far seen in hemophiliacs with AIDS, but a few cases have been reported among Haitian patients. KS is more often seen among New York AIDS cases than those from California or Florida, and is more frequent among white than black patients.

Clinical Manifestation and Course of the Disease

KS is generally believed to be of multifocal origin and, therefore, the new lesions are not the result of metastasis. A male predominance has been reported, with a male-to-female ratio of 15 to 1 in Africa and 3 to 1 in the Memorial Sloan-Kettering series. Of interest is a reversal of the sex ratio in the white population of South African and Algerian cases.

In Africa, lymphadenopathic KS affects mostly youngsters between one and ten years of age. It is rarely seen in the second decade. An increasing incidence of other forms of KS is reported throughout adult life in Africa. The large majority (80 percent) of non-African cases prior to the epidemic of AIDS in 1981 were seen in elderly individuals in the fifth to eighth decades of life. Table 2 summarizes some of the features of classical KS.

In the new epidemic, the average age of the KS cases is reported to be thirty-five. These cases are seen mostly among men, and only very few cases have been noted in women.

In the classical form, Kaposi's sarcoma presents as red-purple macules, plaques, or nodules, mostly on the extremities, but they may appear anywhere in mucous membranes, gastrointestinal tract, and/or skin. Internal organs and especially lymph nodes may be involved. The disease is less frequently seen on the hand, forearm, trunk, head, and neck areas. Solitary lesions on the penis, ear, mouth, eyelid, conjunctiva, and nose have been reported as the sites of initial

Table 2
Classical Kaposi's Sarcoma

Geographical distribution	Eastern Europe, Africa, U.S.A.
Incidence	Africa: 9% all CA U.S.A.: .02–.06/100,000
Male/female	10–15: 1
Age	Average 63 yr. U.S.A.
Clinical type	Africa: 4 types U.S.A.: 3 types

Characteristics

Second primary cancer (lymphoreticular type)
Association with CMV
Association with lowered immunity (renal transplant recipient)
Rare familial cases and lack of association with HLA, A, B, C
Sensitivity of KS to radiation and chemotherapy

manifestation. Other signs and symptoms include pruritus, pain in the lower extremities, and non-pitting edema. Edema of the lower extremities may precede or follow the appearance of the tumor, indicating infiltration of the tumor into the superficial and deep lymphatics. The lesions may coalesce to form large plaques or tumors, which may become eroded, ulcerated, or fungating. New lesions may appear along the superficial vein. Regression of the tumor may occur. KS may appear initially in organs rather than in the skin. Visceral involvement is the pattern most commonly seen in African children, in whom lymphadenopathy is the main clinical feature.

In AIDS patients, KS lesions appear to be elongated and oval-shaped and follow the lines of cleavage as seen in pityriasis rosea. The lesions appear mostly on the upper trunk, head and neck, and upper extremities. Frequent involvement of mucous membrane, lymph nodes, and/or intestinal tract is one of the characteristics of the epidemic form of KS. Cases have been reported in which the disease has manifested only in the lymph node of the intestinal tract. Involvement of lungs, liver, pancreas, adrenal gland, spleen, testis, and larynx have been also reported. As part of this immune deficiency, these patients may also present with systemic complaints of fever, weight loss, malaise, and anorexia.

In European and North American cases, because of the diversity of clinical presentation and the paucity of cases, it has been difficult to establish a useful classification. It is worth noting that KS is more aggressive in renal transplant recipients than the classical cases. The lymphadenopathic type of KS, once limited to Africa, is now seen with frequency in the new epidemic.

This classification in African cases, on the other hand, is very practical and comprehensive and accounts for clinical presentation, course and biologic behavior of the disease, frequency of extracutaneous spread, response and therapy, and histologic patterns.

The course of the disease ranges from slow and indolent to rapid and fulminant with dissemination. The average survival time in the American series of classical KS is reported to be eight to thirteen years. However, survival for up to fifty years and cases with spontaneous regression of the tumor are also reported. In the European and American cases, most patients do not die of their KS but may succumb to death due to second primary malignancies or other diseases that befall the elderly.

In the current epidemic of AIDS, on the other hand, the average survival of KS patients thus far appears to be eighteen months. The course of the disease appears to be aggressive with dissemination and rapid spread. The patients, however, die mostly of opportunistic infections and rarely due to dissemination of KS. The features of both the classical and the new epidemic form of KS are summarized in Table 3.

Histopathology

The disease is thought to start in the dermis and extend upward toward the epidermis. Characteristic histopathologic finding of KS includes interweaving bands of spindle cells and vascular structures embedded in a network of reticular and collagen fibers. The vascular component appears as cleftlike spaces between the spindle cells or delicate capillaries. The spindle cells may show a wide range of nuclear pleomorphism. Other features of KS lesions include extravasated red cells and hemosiderin-laden macrophages as well as lymphocytic infiltration. In general, the histologic features of KS vary according to the quantity of the vascular component, spindle cells, fibrosis, and nuclear pleomorphism in the tumor.

The histologic features of KS seen in the epidemic of AIDS have been reported to be similar to those of classical KS.

Table 3
Kaposi's Sarcoma, Classical Form and the New Outbreak

	Classical KS	*New Outbreak*
Mean age	63	39
Sex ratio (M:F)	10–15:1	all men
Geographic distribution	Africa, Europe, U.S.A.	New York, California
Skin lesions	primarily lower extremities	head, upper extremities, trunk
Lymphadenopathy	rare except African children	frequent
Gastrointestinal lesions	rare	frequent
Course	indolent	aggressive
Associated conditions	second primary malignancies	opportunistic infections
HLA	DR-5 (60%)	DR-5 (60%)

Cell of Origin

The nature of the cell involved in KS is still unknown. A variety of different cell types have been suspected but most studies to date have produced controversial results. The possible reticuloendothelial origin of KS is supported by the increased association of KS with other lymphoreticular malignancies. A more widely accepted view is the endothelial nature of the cell of origin in KS. This view is supported by the recent work of Guarda et al. and Friedman-Kien et al., which demonstrates that the KS cells react with anti–Factor VIII antibodies. It has been shown that endothelial cells and platelets are the source of secretion of Factor VIII.

It is generally believed that KS is a malignant neoplasm. The rarity of documented cases exhibiting metastasis and failure of KS to grow in tissue culture or in laboratory animals is used to argue against a malignant nature for this disease. On the other hand, the aggressive nature of the disease in African children and in homosexual men speaks in favor of its being malignant. One may speculate that KS is a proliferative process of possibly endothelial cells in response to certain stimuli.

Immune Status

Kaposi's sarcoma is a tumor, very sensitive to the normal function of the host immune system. KS has been seen in cases of systemic lupus erythematosus during immunosuppressive therapy and in patients with disorders of the immune system such as immune deficiencies, plasma cell dyscrasia, thymoma, polymyositis, and temporal arteritis. Regression of KS nodules has been reported following decrease or discontinuation of immunosuppressive therapy. In addition, KS has been reported in renal transplant recipients following immunosuppressive therapy. These observations clearly suggest a close association between the host immune system and development of KS. Occurrence of second primary malignancies in KS also suggests a possible role for the immune system in Kaposi's sarcoma.

Master and his co-workers have demonstrated the presence of severe impairment of delayed hypersensitivity reactions to dinitrochlorobenzene in patients with the florid type of KS. In contrast, normal responsiveness was observed in patients with the more benign nodular form of KS. Similar correlation between cell-mediated immunity and clinical morphology of the disease has been described by Taylor and his co-workers. Using *in vitro* lymphocyte responsiveness, it has been shown that patients with the aggressive form of KS had lowered reaction to their own tumor cells as compared to those with the indolent form of disease.

In the epidemic form of KS in homosexual men, progressive and severe immune deficiency is the hallmark of the disease. The deficiency includes: decreased white blood cell count and lymphopenia; imbalance of T lymphocyte subsets with reversal of ratio of T helper/T suppressor cells; decreased responsiveness to mitogens and antigens; decreased level of production of interferon and interleukin 2 by the peripheral blood cells of these patients; and high levels of circulating immune complexes. As a result of this immune dysfunction, the victims of AIDS have developed disseminated and aggressive KS, fatal opportunistic infections, or both. These observations might be taken as evidence relating immune dysfunction with the pathogenesis of KS.

Genetic Predisposition

Cluster occurrence in endemic areas suggests that genetic factors might play a role in KS. The rarity of familial cases negates the possibility of simple Mendelian dominant and recessive inheritance, unless one postulates that a high proportion of incomplete penetrance is involved. On the other hand, studies of major histocompatibility antigens have demonstrated increased frequency of HLA-DR-5 (one of the polymorphic cell-surface markers) in both classical KS and in the new epidemic form of KS. These data suggest a predisposing role for the genetic host factors. In the epidemic of AIDS, similar studies in patients who have only opportunistic infections have not as yet demonstrated any specific increase or decrease in the frequency of HLA antigens. Increase in HLA-DR-5 has also been seen in scleroderma, rheumatoid arthritis, renal cell carcinoma, and mycosis fungoides.

Associated Disorders

Several reviews have described the close association of KS with other diseases. Moertel reported development of KS as a second primary cancer in 51 of 565 cases of lymphoreticular tumors. In another series, only 2 cases of KS were observed among 4,475 cases of lymphoreticular neoplasms. Lymphoreticular malignancies as second primary cancer have also been reported in KS. In one study, 5 cases were observed in a series of 70 KS cases, and in other review, 9 out of 63 cases developed lymphoreticular disorders.

A review from Memorial Sloan-Kettering's cases have shown 34 of 92 KS patients to have had at least one other primary cancer. Of these patients, 58 percent had a second primary malignancy involving the lymphoreticular system. Other cancers seen in association with KS included cancer of the breast, skin, and intestinal tract. Table 4 lists various cancers and other disorders so far seen in the epidemic of AIDS.

Table 4

Epidemic Form of KS-AIDS
Spectrum of Diseases

Kaposi's sarcoma
Opportunistic infections
Non-Hodgkin's lymphoma
Squamous cell carcinoma
Unexplained generalized lymphadenopathy
Progressive wasting syndrome
Autoimmune thrombocytopenia
Progressive multifocal leukoencephalopathy
Nephrotic syndrome

Diabetes mellitus has also been reported to have occurred more frequently in KS patients. Hurlburt and Lincoln reported diabetes mellitus in 6 of 13 cases. DiGiovanna and Safai have reported 16 cases of diabetes mellitus in a series of 90 KS patients. Anemia is also among other diseases reported in association with KS.

Etiology

The cause of KS is still unknown. It is, however, widely believed that a multifactorial etiology is involved in KS. The cluster occurrence of the disease suggests involvement of environmental factors, genetic predisposition, and infectious agents. Several observations suggest geographic and environmental factors do play a role in KS. In the Memorial Sloan-Kettering series (DiGiovanna), 54 out of 77 patients whose places of birth were known were born in endemic areas, suggesting the influence of geography or heritage. However, 6 of the 13 who were born in the United States were known to be of Jewish heritage, thus indicating the influence of heredity rather than geography. The same author reports KS in two brothers, one born in Russia, an endemic area, the other born in the United States. These observations suggest hereditary factors to be more important than geographic variation and that heredity may play a role in the development of KS. This view is further supported by the observation of the increased frequency of HLA-DR-5 in patients with both the classical and epidemic forms of KS.

As for the infectious cause, Giraldo and collaborators have demonstrated herpes-type viral particles in tissue culture lines of KS patients. Furthermore, a close serological association between CMV and KS in European and American cases was demonstrated. CMV-DNA sequences have also been shown in tumor tissues obtained from KS tumors. A high incidence of CMV infection is also reported in other high risk groups, namely the renal transplant recipients and homosexuals. These observations clearly indicate a close association between the CMV and KS and suggest a possible role for CMV in KS. Based on these observations one may speculate that repeated and persistent infections with CMV in genetically predisposed individuals who have some degree of immune disbalance may result in development of KS (Figure 2).

FIGURE 2

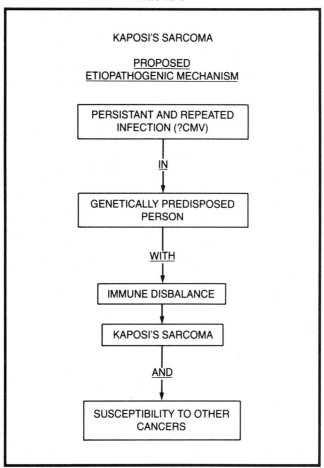

KAPOSI'S SARCOMA

PROPOSED
ETIOPATHOGENIC MECHANISM

PERSISTANT AND REPEATED
INFECTION (?CMV)

IN

GENETICALLY PREDISPOSED
PERSON

WITH

IMMUNE DISBALANCE

KAPOSI'S SARCOMA

AND

SUSCEPTIBILITY TO OTHER
CANCERS

Therapeutic Approach

Although the malignant nature of KS is not as yet documented, this tumor appears to be very sensitive to both radiation and chemotherapy. Radiation therapy has been the most widely used type of treatment for localized disease. In the more aggressive and disseminated form of the disease, however, and in the endemic areas where X-ray therapy facilities are not available, chemotherapy has been the main treatment.

Radiation therapy doses as low as a few hundred rads have been effective for localized tumors. In general early lesions are more radio-sensitive than the older ones. Since the disease is multifocal and recurrent, localized radiation therapy inevitably causes dosimetric problems at multiple junction points. Thus, hemibody radiation, total or subtotal skin electron beam therapy, has been elected in more widespread forms of KS. Holecek et al. utilized extended field radiation therapy (800 rads single dose) and obtained complete responses in 9 of 11 patients. They used Co-60 or 2.5 MeV X ray to parallel opposed fields with a portal size of half a limb. Five recurrences were observed among the 9 complete responders. Nisce and collaborators at Memorial Hospital using total or subtotal skin electron beam irradiation have reported complete responses in 17 of 20 treated cases. Only 2 of the 7 complete responders relapsed in 36 and 43 months of follow-up. Complete responses lasting from 11 to 92 months with a mean of 48 months were observed. This approach is especially effective for patients with widespread skin lesions. Holecek and co-workers reported successful treatment of a patient with a single dose of 800 rads given to the lower half of the body using Co-60 followed six weeks later with a similar dose to the upper half of the body. This was complicated by moderate hematologic and pulmonary toxicity, which cleared subsequently in four months. Goldman has reported successful results with laser irradiation.

In Africa chemotherapy has been widely used. Intralesional infusion of nitrogen mustard was reported by Cook in 75 KS cases in Uganda. He has observed up to 60 percent improvement but with a short-lived remission. Kyalwazi has treated 21 patients with an alkylating agent trenimon, and has reported complete regression in 11 and partial in 9 patients. Two of his patients remained in complete remission for 2 years. Olweny et al. have used Razoxane or ICRF 159 with limited success. A three-drug combination of actinomycin-D, DTIC, and vincristine has been the most effective therapy in more aggressive forms of KS. The three drugs combined was more effective than actinomycin-D alone or in combination with vinblastine. Vincristine has also been tried locally with satisfactory results by Odom and Goette. Bleomycin and BCNU have also been used with considerable clinical activity. A child with aggressive KS has been reported from Italy to have been cured using peptichemo. Cyclophosphamide has been shown to be ineffective in the treatment of KS; in fact, KS has been reported in renal transplant recipients following immunosuppressive therapy with imuran, cyclophosphamide, and/or prednisone.

Other treatment used in KS include methotrexate, topical application of dinitrochlorobenzene, and intralesional injections of PPD (purified protein derivative) or candida extract.

In the epidemic form of KS, combination or single agent chemotherapy has been reported to produce complete or partial responses. However, the patients have usually died of opportunistic infections. VP 16 (etoposide: NSC-141540) which is 4'-dimethyl-epipodaphyllotoxin-3-D-ethylidene glucoside, has been used in the epidemic form of KS and has been reported to produce a high percentage of complete responses (Linda Laubenstein, personal communication).

In early days of the AIDS epidemic it became clear to us that the major problem of patients with the epidemic form of KS is immune deficiency. Furthermore, because of our previous work on the close association of CMV and KS we had the impression that a viral infection might be involved in both AIDS and KS. Thus, at Memorial Hospital we decided to take a different approach and directed our therapeutic approach to the host rather than to the tumor (Kaposi's sarcoma). The biologic response-modifying agents available to date include: interferon, thymic hormones (thymosin, thymopoietin, facteur thymique serique), transfer factor, and mixed bacterial vaccine. Other agents such as MER, BCG and anti-T cell monoclonal antibodies, and interleukin II also could be classified here.

Interferons are a family of biological substances produced by the mammalian cells in response to stimulation by viruses or some other agents. The anti-viral activity of interferons is well documented. In addition, it has been shown that interferons are occasionally capable of inhibiting the growth of some tumors and that under certain conditions interferons may augment immunologic responsiveness. We felt that interferon treatment was worth exploring in the treatment of the epidemic form of KS, partly because of the evidence that an intact immune system could lead to tumor regression in some cases (especially in those receiving renal transplantation) and partly because of the data suggesting that the major morbidity and mortality in this disease was due not to the tumor per se, but to the associated susceptibility to infection, which could be further compromised by chemotherapeutic agents known to be effective in classical KS. A total of 14 patients with KS were treated as part of a phase I study using recombinant leukocyte A interferon supplied by Hoffman-La Roche. The study was conducted by Drs. P. Real, S. Krown, and H. Oettgen of Memorial Sloan-Kettering Cancer Center. Patients were treated with daily doses of either 36 or 54 million units for 28 days, after which the treatment continued on a three-times-per-week basis unless the disease was progressing. At the end of the study, 12 of the 14 patients entered were evaluable for therapeutic responses, and 5 showed major objective responses (3 complete and 2 partial).

Those three patients with complete responses showed regression of their tumors in skin, lymph nodes, and intestinal tract. They have not developed opportunistic infections or other manifestations of AIDS. Some minor improvements were observed in these patients' immunological profile following treatment with interferon. Complete normalization of immune deficiency has not been seen in any case. The side effects seen in the course of this trial have been those known for interferon, including fever, malaise, headache, etc.; no serious side effect was seen. In a phase II trial using recombinant leukocyte A interferon (Hoffman-La Roche), we have now entered close to 40 other patients. The preliminary results of the phase II trial also appear to be promising, but further work is necessary to critically evaluate the effect of interferon on KS as well as on AIDS.

Conclusion

KS is a potentially interesting model of virus-associated human tumors. There is strong evidence suggesting the cytomegalovirus to be the most likely candidate involved in this disease. Further work is needed to clearly define the role of CMV in KS. Moreover, it is necessary to investigate the origin and nature of the cell involved in KS and determine whether the tumor is a malignant neoplasm or a proliferative process.

It is conceivable that a tumor inducer or promoter continues to operate, causing KS and other second primary malignancies.

KS appears to have a short incubation period, taking advantage of the host immune disbalance to develop in a genetically predisposed person. Further determination of the role of host immunity and the major histocompatibility complexes involved is of utmost importance. While KS skin tumors are quite sensitive to radiation and chemotherapy, cases with internal organ involvement respond very poorly to these modalities and die within a short period of time. Association of KS with other lymphomas and occurrence of KS in renal transplant recipients and in cases of AIDS suggest close association of immune dysfunction and development of KS. Thus, immunotherapeutic approaches might prove to be more effective in the treatment of KS than chemo- and radiation therapy.

Part IV

Implications

The tragedy of AIDS extends beyond the victims described in the clinical section of this book. The observation that AIDS can be transmitted through blood products has caused understandable panic in those whose very lives depend on transfusions. It has equally concerned those who must work daily with the blood and secretions of AIDS patients.

Dr. R. Ben Dawson is presently Director of Blood Banks and Professor of Pathology at the University of Maryland. He has held virtually every important position in the American blood banking field and offers direct counsel in a careful essay.

The legitimate concerns of health personnel for their own safety, particularly when dealing with a potentially fatal disorder of unknown cause, are addressed by Dr. Sydney Finegold, Professor of Medicine at UCLA and President of the Infectious Disease Society of America. He is uniquely qualified for this difficult task for, several years ago, he was responsible for controlling the spread of Legionnaires' disease in one of the largest hospital-based outbreaks recorded. Now he both cares for AIDS patients in California and advises doctors and nurses on protecting their own health in these circumstances.

The sudden outbreak of AIDS has also put tremendous pressures on research scientists. Dr. Donald Francis, of CDC's Division of

Hepatitis and Viral Enteritis at Phoenix, Arizona, is a virologist who has worked in many parts of the world tracking smallpox, hepatitis B, and other fatal infections. He explains here how a researcher approaches his work, and some of the special difficulties of reorienting the research community to deal with an epidemic such as AIDS.

9

The Blood Bank Crisis

R. Ben Dawson, M.D.

The possibility that some blood-borne agent may be involved in AIDS is, obviously, of great concern to Red Cross, community blood centers, and hospital blood bank personnel. A fundamental problem is that, like most of our transfusion-related hepatitis, we don't know that a pathogen is lurking in the blood supply until the person becomes sick and the diagnosis is made. A diagnosis of AIDS, in our present state of ignorance about the disease, is of course very bad news. In fact, only very recently has there been any good news at all about AIDS.

1983 seems to be a turning point. Although this is a subjective observation at the moment, it is, I think, worthwhile noting. By the end of 1982 I was beginning to comment to my colleagues that AIDS was the only condition or phenomena in my twenty-five years of carefully studying and watching medicine that was producing news in the form of another development or report every week, not every several weeks or months, which had been the case with all other events in medicine. However, by the time that 1983 had begun, the seemingly weekly reports from various sources, while continuing to record more and more cases and variations on the broad theme of AIDS, were showing a trend toward useful information.[1]

Hepatitis and Homosexuals

Among the first of the encouraging reports was the assurance that our spanking new hepatitis B vaccine is very, very unlikely to transmit AIDS.[2] The assurance provided by this report, from Maurice R. Hilleman, Ph.D., and Marvin E. Jaffe, M.D., Research and Medical Directors of Merck, Sharpe and Dohme, one of the vaccine producers, has a number of aspects to it that suggest a need to compare AIDS and its populations at risk to the populations who are at risk primarily for hepatitis B. Clearly, the process that Merck and other producers use in making their vaccines includes extensive and thorough purification procedures that are known to inactivate representatives of all known groups of animal viruses. The process relies on both biophysical elimination (by ultracentrifugation of infectious particles) and then three sequentially applied chemical inactivation steps (pepsin at pH 2, 8 molar urea, and formalin 1:4000). After production, each lot of vaccine is inoculated into both human and monkey cell culture systems to demonstrate freedom from detectable viruses. Each lot is then administered to chimpanzees to test for the absence of transmission of hepatitis. However, the source material for the vaccine is almost exclusively the gay male population of some of our major cities, the known "high-rate" hepatitis B antigen carriers. Of course, this is the population group apparently at greatest risk for contracting AIDS, or at least they have accumulated the largest number of cases to date. The clearest picture we can gather at the moment about this possible relationship is that the active gay male is at risk of contracting hepatitis B or AIDS, but that the two conditions are in no other way related, as far as we can tell.

In transfusion medicine it was recognized by the beginning of the current decade that hepatitis B virus (HBV) was no longer the leading cause of transfusion hepatitis. A virus or group of viruses called non-A, non-B hepatitis virus was causing 90 percent of the cases of post-transfusion hepatitis. Drs. Hilleman and Jaffe have reminded us that the HBV vaccine does not transmit the non-A, non-B agent(s) in studies done in susceptible chimps and humans.[3] Whether there is a non-A, non-B hepatitis problem in gay males is uncertain; even if it exists, its relationship to AIDS could only be speculated about. It is important to note that the CDC has identified only one or two cases of AIDS in vaccine recipients.[4] One was in a male homosexual whose diagnosis of Kaposi's sarcoma was made three and a half years after receiving Hepatavax-B[R]. This is among nearly 1.5 million people who

have received HBV vaccine. More specifically, among the 800 homosexually active men who received the vaccine, the one or two cases of
AIDS are the only cases in vaccine recipients to date. There were 11
cases of AIDS (2.4 per 800) reported during the same follow-up of
three and a half years among 3,600 unvaccinated homosexual men in
the same population group. These were excluded from the study
primarily because of evidence of prior HBV infection. Thus, there was
actually a higher rate of AIDS among unvaccinated than among
vaccinated homosexual men. Finally, a high-ranking and respected
official of the FDA's Office of Biologics suggests that those at high risk
of contracting hepatitis B should take the new vaccine, because the
"benefits far outweigh the risks." Further, even though AIDS is very
scary, we must remind ourselves that the HBV vaccine is one of the
most sophisticated, seriously thought out and executed, and most
effective of the dozens of vaccines that have been made within the last
half-century.

Another very reasonable discussion of possible links between AIDS
and the hepatitis vaccine reminds us that hepatitis B afflicts as many as
300,000 people per year in the United States, causing between 100 and
200 deaths. The vaccine is the only one available that can prevent the
occurrence of hepatitis B, and according to the clinical trials is better
than 90 percent effective. Yet again we are reminded by the FDA that
the "whole development of the vaccine using human plasma was based
on the understanding that extraordinary measures would assure that
nothing is transmitted."[5]

Hemophilia

Additional evidence that AIDS is, in part at least, the response to a
blood-borne agent comes from an alarming number of cases in hemophiliacs, who suffer from a fairly uncommon bleeding disorder, and one
case in an infant who had received ordinary blood transfusions. There
are over a dozen cases of AIDS in the 15–18,000 American hemophiliacs, most of whom are maintained with the freeze-dried anti-hemophiliac blood-clotting factor called Factor VIII.[6] This agent is prepared
from lots pooled from tens of thousands of plasma units collected
within the American plasma industry and from Red Cross plasma
salvage programs.

A recent study suggests greater susceptibility to AIDS in hemophiliac patients getting the freeze-dried treatment (LYOPH group), compared to single-donor cryo (CRYO group). Members of the LYOPH

group have greater abnormalities in immunity. These abnormalities in cell-mediated immunity include a relative decrease in helper T cells and an increase in suppressor T cells. There is depressed natural killer activity and diminished lymphocyte proliferative response to stimulation.[7]

One early strategy in the blood banking community, still being considered by many, is switching on a large scale to the use of single blood donor cryoprecipitate units for treating bleeding episodes in hemophiliac patients. The thinking has been that this reduction in the number of donor units a patient is exposed to may reduce the risk of an individual patient receiving the AIDS agent in his therapy. While the thinking is still of merit, it has not been widely acted on.

Transfusion

The CDC in December 1982 reported four and possibly five new hemophilia patients developing AIDS. In all but one case, the individuals were severe hemophiliacs requiring large amounts of clotting factor concentrate. Alarmingly, two of the five new cases of AIDS in hemophiliacs were children whose exposure to the plasma fraction therapies could not have been as long or great. At least one Canadian hemophiliac has AIDS, and in Canada two normal non-immunosuppressed patients got AIDS from blood transfusions from Haitians. The three most recent reports of AIDS in hemophilia patients in the United States are in patients in the central as opposed to coastal states, i.e., not in the gay capital regions. However, many of the plasma centers, from which their anti-hemophiliac factor concentrate material is derived, are located in those large coastal cities.

In December of 1982 a San Francisco infant born to healthy non-Haitian heterosexual parents developed a case of what was said to be AIDS after receiving blood transfusions from nineteen donors to correct an Rh hemolytic disorder. One of the donors, a forty-eight-year-old male, had been in good health at the time of the blood donation, but began to develop AIDS symptoms eight months afterward. The diagnosis of AIDS was eventually made and the donor died a year and a half later. To the CDC this report suggests an infectious agent theory of transmission. It also suggests that the agent may be spread many, many months before the donor has any symptoms. Thus, the incubation period may be in the neighborhood of a year (range six months to two years), making case-following extraordinarily difficult and long in terms of developing data.[8]

CDC's case for an infectious agent is supported further by reports in January of 1983 that AIDS may occur in heterosexual or homosexual couples. Two females who have been steady sexual partners of males with AIDS have developed the syndrome. Both females were previously healthy and had no known risk factor other than contact with male partners who eventually developed AIDS. In the same report, the CDC noted that AIDS developed in both members of a homosexual couple in Denmark.[9] AIDS has also occurred after a transfusion in Haiti.[10]

Although people in my field of blood banking and transfusion therapy are downplaying the idea of a blood-borne agent, the CDC is considering a blood-borne virus or agent as a good possibility. The above cited transfusion-related evidence certainly suggests that the syndrome may be blood-borne or infectious. Also, since it seems to follow a pattern—at least in terms of susceptible groups—that is common to that of hepatitis B, the precautions that are recommended and regularly carried out for protection from hepatitis B virus infections would seem to be useful and should be applied for protection when contact with AIDS patients or their body fluids is necessary. Needles and syringes should be handled as stipulated specifically in section A of the *Morbidity and Mortality Weekly Report* of CDC, November 1982. Also, the usual extra precautions of changing laboratory coats and gowns, regular handwashing, and the use of gloves are all mentioned. Not specifically mentioned is the practice advocated in Great Britain for protection from hepatitis, that of wearing double gloves. Additional recommendations for laboratory precautions are recommended and outlined.[11]

Transfusion Therapy

Transfusion therapy in the United States results from over 10 million blood donations a year. These supply approximately 3 million Americans with transfusions, usually for surgery. However, almost 20,000 hemophiliacs are frequently receiving blood products or derivatives. If AIDS were rampant in the nation's blood banks, the CDC reasons, there would be more cases. "For the average person who needs to get a transfusion, it is no concern," says Jaffe of the CDC, "but all of these recent cases together make us feel strongly that this is an issue that needs to be re-reviewed."[12] However, AIDS does have a very long incubation period and thus it is possible that it could be rampant in our blood banks but not yet revealing itself in patients.

The December 1982 meeting of the Advisory Committee of the Office of Biologics of the FDA in Bethesda with blood-banking and Red Cross blood program directors was primarily informative, with no strong recommendations being made. However, in January of 1983 a meeting between commercial blood bankers and government health officials resulted in two definite suggestions: not allowing gays or Haitians to donate, and screening donors for past infections of hepatitis B on the presumption that the people who get hepatitis might get AIDS.

The plasma industry and commercial blood banks, represented by their American Blood Resources Association (ABRA), should be commended for taking the firm stand, in January of 1983, of questioning their donors and disqualifying those from high-risk groups. On the other hand, the other big suppliers of blood and plasma, the American Red Cross (ARC) and the American Association of Blood Banks (AABB) are encouraging voluntary disqualification by members of the high-risk groups. It seems no longer prudent to deny the extremely high likelihood of AIDS being transmitted as a blood-borne agent. Thus, a strong stand with respect to blood and plasma donors seems warranted.

Supporting the theory or proposal of a blood-borne agent are the cases of the women victims who are sexual partners of men with AIDS, and the group of children. So far 26 children less than five years old appear to have had the syndrome and 10 have died. None had Kaposi's, but they have had pneumocystis and other infections characteristic of immune system breakdowns. They are similar in that respect to the Haitian adults. Indeed, most of the children's parents are Haitians, IV drug users, or have had homosexual contact. Some of the parents have AIDS and others could be carriers.

Kaposi's sarcoma in Africa is linked to a viral infection caused by the cytomegalovirus (CMV). CMV infection or infestation is considered a sexually transmitted disease (STD) and most gay men carry one form or another of CMV, usually with flulike symptoms. Pre-dating AIDS and apparently unrelated to sexually transmitted disease is the known occurence of CMV in transfused blood units. The virus is not a strong or virulent disease producer, so attempts by blood banks up to now to detect it have been limited to protection of the immunodeficient or immuno-compromised patient.

An interesting, although very speculative possibility is for a CMV-like agent (perhaps a virulent mutation) to have been picked up in Africa and transited through Haiti, where it was picked up by visiting

Americans for transport on to the United States. In support of this possibility is the contracting of AIDS in infants of Haitian mothers. One of these died with AIDS pneumonia and generalized CMV infection.[13]

Summary

Although the gay population could be screened for the several HBV markers, it may be significant that 90 percent of AIDS victims are also positive in antibody tests for hepatitis B, and 90 percent of Haitians as well have an HBV marker. However, to use such a "surrogate agent" as a marker for AIDS is criticized by Donald Armstrong of Memorial Sloan-Kettering Cancer Center, who said, "I have no doubt that this is an infectious disease. I think we have to find the agent. A surrogate agent isn't good enough."[14] Perhaps it is not good enough, but until we can detect the agent or control the disease, we should use what we have available to protect our patients and personnel at risk from contact, namely: knowledge of high-risk groups and the highly associated markers such as HBV and CMV.

Precautions

To date no AIDS cases have been documented among health care personnel caring for AIDS patients or among laboratory workers processing blood samples. Also, no person-to-person transmission has been identified other than through intimate contact or blood transfusion. But since transmission occurs through these latter routes, the following recommended actions are suggested. This is a composite list from several sources including The American Association of Blood Banks, The American Blood Resources Association, The American Red Cross, and the U.S. Public Health Service.

1. Use infectious precautions when drawing blood or handling tissue specimens from known or suspected AIDS patients. Blood from such patients will be used only for diagnostic or research purposes, not for human transfusions.
2. Refuse as blood donors or plasma donors by direct questioning those with AIDS, with symptoms or signs suggestive of AIDS, or at increased risk of acquiring AIDS. The latter group includes: sexual partners of AIDS patients; sexually active homosexual or bisexual men with multiple partners; Haitians who

have entered the United States since 1978; present or past abusers of intravenous drugs; patients with hemophilia; and sexual partners of individuals at increased risk for AIDS.

3. Symptoms and signs that are suggestive of AIDS include unexplained fevers or weight loss, persistent night sweats, signs of swollen glands, malaise, chronic diarrhea, and signs of Kaposi's sarcoma (pink to purple flat or raised blotches or bumps occuring anywhere on the skin or mucous membranes).

Implementation of these recommendations presently varies from self-exclusion after the donor reads a leaflet describing the risk groups and suggestive signs and symptoms, to direct questioning about the potentially associated factors. An intermediate approach advised by the hospital blood bank association, AABB, is to have donors sign a statement such as: "I have read the literature provided by the blood bank concerning AIDS, and understand that members of certain groups at increased risk have been asked to refrain from donating blood at this time." If direct questioning is not used, then the following, additional statement should be added to the one just above for donors to sign: "I also understand that certain signs and symptoms that are suggestive of AIDS could make my blood potentially harmful to others, if transfused."

☐ I will therefore certify that I am not in a risk group nor do I have suggested signs or symptoms.
☐ I am not sure and/or want my blood used only for research.
☐ I will not donate at this time.

_____
(initials or signature)

If these recommendations are adhered to and we take the additional precaution of testing for HBV and CMV antibody markers, we will have done the best we know how to contain the AIDS agent(s), preventing it from getting into our blood supply.

Finally, we consider this a health problem, not a social or prejudicial problem. We have always refused certain blood donors because of illness, geography, habit, or association. In recommending the above actions, we seek only to prevent the spread of a disease that has already shown itself capable of infecting disparate populations, with deadly result.

10

Protecting Health Personnel

Sydney M. Finegold, M.D.

Protecting people against AIDS is made difficult by many factors. At the present time there is lack of agreement as to what constitutes a case, absence of clear markers for the disease except when it is in an advanced stage, and epidemiologic data suggesting that there is a latent period or incubation period of several months to as long as two years between exposure to AIDS and recognizable clinical illness. The latter, of course, implies that transmission of the disease may occur before the illness is recognizable. The fact that a significant proportion of gay men who are asymptomatic or who have only nonspecific symptoms have altered immune function and that this phenomenon has also been noted in patients with hemophilia suggests that the pool of individuals who may be capable of transmitting the disease could be considerably larger than the presently known number of patients in whom AIDS has been diagnosed.

The epidemiology of AIDS cases resembles that of hepatitis B virus infection, which can be transmitted sexually, by administration of infected blood or blood products, and by skin puncture for other purposes.

Although infectious disease clinicians and epidemiologists rise to the challenge of an outbreak of epidemic, the study of AIDS has been much more than an intellectual challenge. It is rather frightening in that, two years after the first case was reported, the etiology is still unknown and there is no end in sight for this deadly disease. Already more patients have died from AIDS or its complications than from both Legionnaires' disease and toxic shock syndrome. It is small wonder then that the still unknown agent responsible for AIDS is likened to the "Andromeda Strain."

The panic engendered in certain individuals is a little reminiscent of that associated with the bubonic plague centuries ago, even though there were considerably more cases and deaths over a much shorter time span with the plague. The following description of the plague by Giovanni Boccaccio is of interest because of certain parallels.

In the year of our lord [sic] 1348, in Florence, the finest city of all Italy, there occurred a most terrible plague: either because of the influence of the planets or sent from God as a just punishment for our sins, it has broken out some years earlier in the East, and after passing from place to place and wreaking incredible havoc along the way had now reached the West where [it spread], in spite of all the means that art and human foresight could suggest, such as keeping the city clear from filth, and excluding all suspected people. . . . Purple spots appeared in most parts of the body . . . the usual messengers of death. To the cure of this disease, neither the knowledge of medicine nor the power of drugs was of any effect, whether because the disease was itself fatal or because the physicians, whose number was increased by quacks and women pretenders, could discover neither cause nor cure, and so few escaped. The disease grew daily by being communicated from the sick to the well. . . . Nor was it [necessary] to converse or even to come near the sick; even touching their clothes or anything they had touched was sufficient. . . . The events and similar others caused various fears among those people who survived, all tending to the same cruel and uncharitable end which was to avoid the sick and everything that had been near them. . . . Some felt it best to live temperately . . . but others maintained free living and would deny no passion or appetite they wished to gratify. . . . And the public distress was such that all laws, whether human or divine, were ignored.

Responsibility of Medical Personnel to AIDS Patients

AIDS patients, not surprisingly, express guilt, anger, remorse, depression, and despair. Most importantly, there is fear and especially fear of desertion, a worry not unfounded, for an ignorant society has typically cast out its "lepers." It should be appreciated that most homosexual men do not have the support of their families because they do not discuss their life-style with them. AIDS patients, then, may be terrified and need a tremendous amount of support. It is tragic and almost unbelievable to learn that occasionally health-care personnel, including physicians and nurses, have refused to care for AIDS patients. It is reminiscent of the cruel and uncharitable reactions of the Middle Ages. Fortunately, such instances have been rare. On the other hand, there have been gratifying examples of health care personnel volunteering to care for AIDS patients and attempting to obtain innovative in-service educational opportunities and resources for psychiatric and emotional support for these patients. It should be noted that counseling should be done on a one-to-one basis, rather than with groups, because of the risk of transmission of infection.

It is inconceivable that we in the health-care professions, and especially physicians and nurses, could refuse to work with AIDS patients—or any other type of patient for that matter. It has been the tradition of medicine that anyone requiring medical care, regardless of his or her background and regardless of the nature of the disease involved, should receive optimal care. This includes the enemy during wartime, criminals, and the patient with an unknown, possibly dangerous, communicable disease. Our service to humanity must, as Glick has said, rank as a higher priority than personal gratification (and, we might add, personal concern).[1] This characteristic, as Wyngaarden notes, is a reaffirmation of Hippocrates, Osler, and every other truly great physician.[2] Lewis Thomas states, ". . . I do not foresee any real change in the fundamental responsibility of doctors [in relation to changing technology]. . . . I hope that they will be bound by the same deeply personal obligation to serve their patients."[3] The Oath and Prayer of Maimonides is worth recalling: "Thy Eternal providence has appointed me to watch over the life and health of Thy creatures. . . . May I never see in the patient anything but a fellow creature in pain. . . . Grant energy unto both body and the Soul that I might e'er unhindered ready be to mitigate the woes, sustain and help the rich and poor, the good and bad, enemy and friend. O let me e'er behold in the afflicted and suffering, only the human being." It is interesting to note that a presidential commission set up to investigate health care in the face of our present budget cutbacks and fiscal austerity concluded that society has an "ethical obligation to ensure equitable access to health care" for *all* Americans.

It is important to recognize that, to date, there has been no instance of transmission of AIDS to health workers or to laboratory personnel. Nevertheless, what we know about the transmission of the disease indicates that their concern is a valid one. It clearly would be wise to keep certain personnel who might be at extra risk, such as immunosuppressed or pregnant individuals, from working with AIDS patients, but the vast majority of personnel should regard it as their duty to care for these unfortunate patients.

Obviously, there is also a responsibility *to* health care providers for a commitment of society's resources. We must work quickly to obtain the needed answers concerning questions of transmissibility, degree of risk under various conditions, and the cause, cure, and prevention of AIDS.

Protection of Medical Personnel and of Other Patients

At present, the risk to hospital personnel, if any, cannot be judged. Certainly the risk of acquiring the disease is much greater in bathhouses than in hospitals. As with hepatitis, there are undoubtedly unknown exposures in everyday society. The epidemiology of AIDS appears similar to that of hepatitis B; studies on hepatitis B have shown that emergency ward nurses, blood bank personnel, and laboratory technicians are at the greatest risk, followed by staff of the department of pathology, IV teams, surgical housestaff, and intensive care unit nurses. Health care providers at moderate risk (relatively) would include medical housestaff, general ward nurses, and dietitians. Once again, it should be noted that, to date, there have been no cases of AIDS documented among health care or laboratory personnel related to taking care of AIDS patients or processing their specimens. Furthermore, to date there has been no person-to-person transmission identified other than through intimate contact or by transfusion of blood products.

The Centers for Disease Control (CDC) has published suggested precautions to be observed by clinical and laboratory staffs dealing with AIDS patients or suspected AIDS patients. The basic principle underlying these suggested precautions is for clinical and laboratory personnel to avoid direct contact of their own skin and mucous membranes with blood, blood products, excretions, secretions, and tissues of persons judged likely to have AIDS. In this connection, it is most discouraging to note a recent study in which it was found that in two medical intensive care units physicians washed their hands only 28 percent of the time following patient contact.[4] The precautions, which are listed below, do not address outpatient care, dental care, surgery, autopsy, or hemodialysis specifically. CDC recommends that hospitals and laboratories adapt the precautions to their individual circumstances.

    A. The following precautions are advised in providing care to AIDS patients:

        1. Extraordinary care must be taken to avoid accidental wounds from sharp instruments contaminated with potentially infectious material and to avoid contact of open skin lesions with material from AIDS patients.

        2. Gloves should be worn when handling blood specimens, blood-soiled items, body fluids, excretions, and secretions, as well as surface, materials, and objects exposed to them.

        3. Gowns should be worn when clothing may be soiled with body fluids, blood, secretions, or excretions.

        4. Hands should be washed after removing gowns and gloves and before leaving the rooms of known or suspected AIDS patients. Hands should also be washed thoroughly and immediately if they become contaminated with blood.

        5. Blood and other specimens should be labeled prominently with a special warning, such as "Blood Precautions" or "AIDS Precautions." If the outside of the specimen container is visibly contaminated with blood, it should be cleaned with a disinfectant (such as a 1:10 dilution of 5.25% sodium hypochlorite [household bleach] with water). All blood specimens should be placed in a second container, such as an impervious bag, for transport. The container or bag should be examined carefully for leaks or cracks.

        6. Blood spills should be cleaned up promptly with disinfectant solution, such as sodium hypochlorite (see above).

7. Articles soiled with blood should be placed in an impervious bag prominently labled "AIDS Precautions" or "Blood Precautions" before being sent for reprocessing or disposal. Alternatively, such contaminated items may be placed in plastic bags of a particular color designated solely for disposal of infectious wastes by the hospital. Disposable items should be incinerated or disposed of in accord with the hospital's policies for disposal of infectious wastes. Reusable items should be reprocessed in accord with hospital policies for hepatitis B virus–contaminated items. Lensed instruments should be sterilized after use on AIDS patients.

8. Needles should not be bent after use, but should be promptly placed in a puncture-resistant container used solely for such disposal. Needles should not be reinserted into their original sheaths before being discarded into the container, since this is a common cause of needle injury.

9. Disposable syringes and needles are preferred. Only needle-locking syringes or one-piece needle-syringe units should be used to aspirate fluids from patients, so that collected fluid can be safely discharged through the needle, if desired. If reusable syringes are employed, they should be decontaminated before reprocessing.

10. A private room is indicated for patients who are too ill to use good hygiene, such as those with profuse diarrhea, fecal incontinence, or altered behavior secondary to central nervous system infections.

Precautions appropriate for particular infections that concurrently occur in AIDS patients should be added to the above, if needed.

B. The following precautions are advised for persons performing laboratory tests or studies on clinical specimens or other potentially infectious materials (such as inoculated tissue cultures, embryonated eggs, animal tissues, etc.) from known or suspected AIDS cases:

1. Mechanical pipetting devices should be used for the manipulation of all liquids in the laboratory. Mouth pipetting should not be allowed.

2. Needles and syringes should be handled as stipulated in Section A (above).

3. Laboratory coats, gowns, or uniforms should be worn while working with potentially infectious materials and should be discarded appropriately before leaving the laboratory.

4. Gloves should be worn to avoid skin contact with blood, specimens containing blood, blood-soiled items, body fluids, excretions, and secretions, as well as surfaces, materials, and objects exposed to them.

5. All procedures and manipulations of potentially infectious material should be performed carefully to minimize the creation of droplets and aerosols.

6. Biological safety cabinets (Class I or II) and other primary containment devices (e.g., centrifuge safety cups) are advised whenever procedures are conducted that have a high potential for creating aerosols or infectious droplets. These include centrifuging, blending, sonicating, vigorous mixing, and harvesting infected tissues from animals or embryonated eggs. Fluorescent activated cell sorters generate droplets that could potentially result in infectious aerosols. Translucent plastic shielding between the droplet-collecting area and the equipment operator should be used to reduce the presently uncertain magnitude of this risk. Primary containment devices are also used in handling materials that might contain concentrated infectious agents or organisms in greater quantities than expected in clinical specimens.

7. Laboratory work surfaces should be decontaminated with a disinfectant, such as sodium hypochlorite solution, following any spill of potentially infectious material and at the completion of work activities.

8. All potentially contaminated materials used in laboratory tests should be decontaminated, preferably by autoclaving, before disposal or reprocessing.

9. All personnel should wash their hands following com-

pletion of laboratory activities, removal of protective clothing, and before leaving the laboratory.

C. The following additional precautions are advised for studies involving experimental animals inoculated with tissues or other potentially infectious materials from individuals with known or suspected AIDS.

1. Laboratory coats, gowns, or uniforms should be worn by personnel entering rooms housing inoculated animals. Certain nonhuman primates, such as chimpanzees, are prone to throw excreta and to spit at attendants; personnel attending inoculated animals should wear molded surgical masks and goggles or other equipment sufficient to prevent potentially infective droplets from reaching the mucosal surfaces of their mouths, nares, and eyes. In addition, when handled, other animals may disturb excreta in their bedding. Therefore, the above precautions should be taken when handling them.

2. Personnel should wear gloves for all activities involving direct contact with experimental animals and their bedding and cages. Such manipulations should be performed carefully to minimize the creation of aerosols and droplets.

3. Necropsy of experimental animals should be conducted by personnel wearing gowns and gloves. If procedures generating aerosols are performed, masks and goggles should be worn.

4. Extraordinary care must be taken to avoid accidental sticks or cuts with sharp instruments contaminated with body fluids or tissues of experimental animals inoculated with material from AIDS patients.

5. Animal cages should be decontaminated, preferably by autoclaving, before further cleaning and washing.

6. Only needle-locking syringes or one-piece needle-syringe units should be used to inject potentially infectious fluids into experimental animals.

The above precautions are intended to apply to both clinical and research laboratories. Biological safety cabinets and other safety equipment may not be generally available in clinical laboratories. Assistance should be sought from a microbiology laboratory, as needed, to assure containment facilities are adequate to permit laboratory tests to be conducted safely.

Some individuals have been unwilling to use masks or gowns for fear of enhancing the anxiety that already exists with regard to this syndrome. At the UCLA Medical Center the option for personnel to use masks if the patient is coughing or to wear gowns if the patient is soiled has been very helpful in obtaining good cooperation from all health care personnel.[5] Prior to the availability of this option, there had been some reluctance on the part of some health care personnel to deal with AIDS patients. At UCLA, precautions for outpatients are generally consistent with what has been recommended by CDC for inpatients. When possible, patients with AIDS are seen in designated examination rooms on designated days. Having these patients remain in waiting rooms with patients who may be severely immunocompromised is avoided. When possible, vital signs are obtained and all treatments conducted in the examination rooms. Whenever possible, patients with cough or diarrhea are admitted directly to the examination rooms. In the case of AIDS patients requiring surgery, the patient goes directly to the operating room rather than to a pre-op room first. Surgery on such patients is scheduled for the end of the day, when possible, to permit adequate time for thorough cleanup following the procedure. "Contaminated technique" is followed in the operating room and a filter is used in the anesthesia equipment. The patient is returned to a private room, rather than to the recovery room. All specimens for the laboratory from AIDS patients are handled in the main laboratory; none is handled in any ward laboratory. When possible, a disposable proctoscope or a separate proctoscope or other endoscope is used exclusively for AIDS patients. When this is not possible, appropriate disinfection, as employed for instruments used on patients with hepatitis B, is considered adequate. AIDS patients requiring critical care nursing are placed in private rooms. Although the physician is responsible for informing the nursing staff that the patient has AIDS, or possibly has AIDS, and ordering appropriate isolation or precautions, the nursing staff is encouraged to check the patient's diagnosis and place the patient in isolation if it is appropriate and has not been ordered.

At the San Francisco General Hospital,[6] plans are being drafted to establish a central unit to provide care for AIDS patients. Instead of having these patients scattered and in private rooms throughout the hospital, their location in a central unit would offer some attractive advantages for staff as well as for patients. In such a unit it would be easier to educate a hand-picked, concerned staff who could provide better care for patients. Psychological support services for patients, patients' families, and staff—whether provided by the hospital or by

community groups—could be more readily available. Uniform isolation practices can be taught and enforced more readily in a dedicated
unit. The serious nature of AIDS and the high fatality rate has
produced concern among workers at the hospital. This concern can
best be handled by an educational program set up by a clinical nurse
specialist or nurse instructor working from a central unit in association
with the attending physicians. Ready access to someone who can
answer questions and organize educational programs will help alleviate
concern. Provision should be made for a minor procedure room for
bronchoscopy and endoscopy of AIDS patients. Special precautions
required for protection of operators can thus be carried out more
effectively. Decontamination of instruments can be better controlled.

The AIDS central unit at the San Francisco General Hospital would
be made up of a number of private rooms, each with a sink and toilet.
Knee action sinks for handwashing would be provided at the entrance
to the unit, in two additional locations in the main hallway, and in each
patient room. The procedure room for bronchoscopy and other endoscopy would be maintained under negative pressure. Decontamination
facilities would be nearby. Well-trained phlebotomists with sufficient
time to work carefully would be provided. Respirators used for AIDS
patients would have disposable tubing. Segments that may be contaminated would be sterilized, using either ethylene oxide or glutaralde-
hyde. Goggles would be worn when any splatter is expected; careful
handwashing after patient contact would be stressed even when gloves
have been worn.

Machine isolation should be provided for dialysis unit patients.
Each AIDS or possible AIDS patient should be in a separate room
since even two AIDS patients with apparently identical opportunisitic
infections may be infected with organisms with significant strain
differences.

Blood banking procedures have been discussed in detail in the
chapter by Dr. Dawson. These are clearly of the utmost importance.
Included are such considerations as physicians applying strict medical
indications for transfusions, the use of autologous blood transfusions
when feasible, more careful screening of blood donors, the need for
studies to evaluate screening procedures for their effectiveness in
identifying and excluding blood and plasma with a high probability of
transmitting AIDS, and continued study toward development of safer
blood products for use by hemophilia patients. Various organizations
have proposed different methods for screening of individuals at increased risk for AIDS to avoid their donating blood or plasma. The

American Association of Physicians for Human Rights is a national organization dedicated to unprejudiced and well-informed medical care for gay and lesbian patients. This group feels that testing for previous hepatitis B infection (by antibody to hepatitis B core antigen) and measuring the absolute lymphocyte count are probably the best indicators of blood that may be at high risk for carrying an AIDS agent.

It would seem prudent for dentists and dental technicians to wear gloves and a mask when working on AIDS patients or possible AIDS patients.

It is important that pathologists and morticians be made aware of the possibility or definite presence of AIDS in connection with examination of biopsy specimens, performance of autopsies, and embalming. Both of these groups should also be informed about any communicable disease that may be present in such patients.

Protection of Subjects at Risk for AIDS

Sexual contact with known or suspected AIDS patients should be avoided. Since the syndrome is more prevalent among sexually active homosexual men, persons in this group can reduce their risk by minimizing the number of their sexual contacts, avoiding those who are sexually promiscuous, and avoiding all casual and anonymous contacts. The average number of lifetime sexual contacts among promiscuous gays with AIDS has been reported to be over 1,000. These individuals frequent homosexual bars and bathhouses (where a typical visit may include sex with several deliberately anonymous men). Many of these individuals use "poppers" (inhaled amyl or butyl nitrite), drugs that are said to enhance orgasm. Patients should emphasize to their sex contacts that they must not bring any new diseases home with them. Some physicians urge patients to eliminate anal intercourse, which may result in bleeding or trauma to the mucosa and is a possible source of transmission of AIDS. Some advise their gay patients to use condoms. It has also been suggested that gays should attempt to find alternative means of socializing and of meeting new partners, avoiding casual contacts and learning more about their future sex partner.

The American Association of Physicians for Human Rights has a number of specific suggestions to reduce the risk of acquiring AIDS. The two major steps that they stress are to decrease the number of different partners with whom one has sex, thus avoiding men who have many different sex partners. Secondly, they advise not injecting any drugs not prescribed and avoiding sexual contact with IV drug users. This organization states that certain sexual practices are known to be associated with an increased risk of sexually transmitted diseases and that reducing these factors may decrease the risk of AIDS. Included are: 1) one-time encounters with anonymous partners and/or group sex; 2) oral-anal contact ("rimming"); 3) "fisting" (both giving and receiving); 4) active or passive rectal intercourse (use of condoms may be helpful); 5) fecal contamination through scatological sex. The organization notes that an additional probable risk factor may be mucous membrane (mouth or rectum) contact with semen or urine.

Further suggestions are: 1) to know your sex partner and ask about his health and when in doubt, reconsider; 2) shower before sex and inspect your partner; 3) take care of your general health (get adequate rest, good nutrition, physical exercise, reduce stress, and reduce toxic substances such as alcohol, cigarettes, marijuana, "poppers," and non-prescription drugs). I would also urge homosexuals who know or suspect that they have any transmissible disease not to risk the health of others.

To help homosexuals recognize the possibility of AIDS in contacts, the American Association of Physicans for Human Rights provides the following list of symptoms or indications of AIDS:

1. Swollen glands (enlarged lymph nodes, with or without pain, usually in the neck, armpits, or groin) lasting for more than one month.
2. Pink to purple flat or raised blotches or bumps, usually painless, occurring on or under the skin, inside the mouth, nose, eyelids, or rectum. Initially, they may look like bruises that do not go away, and they are usually harder than the skin around them.
3. Persistent white spots or unusual blemishes in the mouth.
4. Weight loss that is unexpected and greater than approximately ten pounds in less than two months.
5. Drenching night sweats that may occur on and off and last at least several weeks.
6. Cough and shortness of breath (a persistent and often dry cough that is not from smoking and has lasted too long to be from a common respiratory infection).
7. Fever (an elevation of temperature above 99°F.) that has persisted for more than ten days.
8. Diarrhea (persistent and not explained by other causes).

One may also wonder about the risk involved in the practices among some gays of ear piercing, nipple piercing, and tattooing.

Marmor and colleagues reported an interesting study of 20 homosexual men with confirmed Kaposi's sarcoma and 40 controls. Two risk factors were felt to be highly significant in this study. One was the use of amyl nitrite (an average of 542 lifetime uses of this compound among the Kaposi's sarcoma patients) and the other was the number of sex partners per month (an average of 10 per month in Kaposi's sarcoma patients).

The predictive value of T cell typing and function testing is still being evaluated. It is not appropriate that this type of test be used at this time for clinical screening.

Protection of AIDS Patients

Certainly the factors suggested as offering protection to subjects at risk for AIDS (changes in sexual practices and avoidance of various drugs) are also advisable for patients with AIDS. Other immunosuppressive drugs such as corticosteroids should be avoided whenever possible. Patients with AIDS should not work in hospital environments, where they would be exposed to many unusual and virulent pathogens. When such subjects are hospitalized, some degree of "reverse" or "protective" isolation would be desirable. There would not appear to be any role for cotrimoxazole prophylaxis against *Pneumocystis* pneumonia, although it would possibly be useful in preventing recurrences.

Protection of Others from AIDS Patients

The protection of other patients from AIDS patients in the hospital setting has already been discussed in the section dealing with isolation procedures. Pregnant women should also avoid contact with AIDS patients because of the risk of infection with cytomegalovirus, as well as the risk of AIDS itself.

AIDS patients should not donate blood nor should they donate organs. It would seem prudent to ask that AIDS patients not engage in food preparation or handling for others, particularly if they have an intestinal infection.

It is to be hoped that AIDS patients would forego sexual intercourse out of consideration for their contacts. Some AIDS patients have adopted this practice already.

What Should Our Priorities for Research Be?

1. Search for the etiologic agent and for any "collaborating" agents and/or drugs.
   a. Appropriate body fluids and tissues should be injected into primates, including rhesus monkeys.
   b. Pursue further studies of the naturally occurring disease similar to AIDS that afflicts rhesus monkeys.
   c. When an etiologic agent is identified, determine its susceptibility to various inactivating agents.
2. Prospective clinical and laboratory studies (including viral cultures and serologies) of people at high risk of developing AIDS and of those with incompletely developed Acquired Immune Deficiency Syndrome. This would probably best be done as a case-control study. Such a study should yield a better definition of AIDS and better early markers of the disease.
3. Determine more fully the relative risk of different specific types of sexual activity, drug usage, and other aspects of life-style.
4. Develop screening procedures to identify blood and plasma with a high probability of transmitting AIDS.
5. Monitoring of those exposed to persons with AIDS (including health care professionals).
6. Continuing evaluation of hepatitis B vaccine recipients is needed to provide more definitive answers regarding the safety of the vaccine (as far as AIDS is concerned).
7. Studies of various modes of therapy for AIDS and its complicating infections are needed. Ultimately, we would hope to develop preventive measures.

11

The Search for the Cause

Donald P. Francis, M.D.

From the time of the initial reports of AIDS, speculation began regarding the cause of this unique disease. There have been proponents from various camps. Some were convinced that AIDS sprang from today's modern environment with its chemicals or drugs; others favored the theory of an infectious agent that has circulated since antiquity. Some believe there are multiple causes that, because of the complexity of modern life, have been allowed to come together, while others think there is a single cause that by chance was brought to modern man from distant lands.

How can such disparate proposals be eventually united to help direct the search for the cause? Hypothesis by hypothesis, piece by piece, each is tested. But following these various hunches is expensive, requiring personnel time and logistical support. Thus, the search cannot be a random, helter-skelter approach. Instead, efforts must be directed toward the most likely hypothesis. As one hunch is developed, so is a test by which it can be proven or disproven. If the initial tests are passed, others are developed and the next hypothesis is tested. And so on, until either a dead-end is reached, a negative answer is found, or the cause is discovered.

Before any search for a cause could begin, however, an agreement was needed regarding what was to be considered a "case" of this new disease. After all, was a "case" someone found to have enlarged lymph nodes or was a "case" someone who had died of Kaposi's sarcoma? Some working definition, however arbitrary, was required. With time and knowledge, this definition could be modified, but a starting point was mandatory. With the help of the clinicians who took care of AIDS patients, CDC physicians arrived at a case definition from which subsequent epidemiologic and laboratory investigations grew. The presumption was that there was a single disease of the immune system that became clinically apparent in multiple ways. A "case" of AIDS was defined as anyone under the age of sixty with Kaposi's sarcoma and anyone (regardless of age) with a severe opportunistic infection without any underlying cause (such as cancer, chemotherapy, etc.).

Using this definition, analyses could be made of AIDS occurrence. A picture was drawn of an epidemic disease that was initially reported as affecting only homosexual men but was soon discovered in a wide range of groups including sexual partners (homosexual and heterosexual) of patients, people who received blood or blood products from others (intravenous drug users, hemophiliacs, and recipients of transfusions), infants and children who were born to or lived with some of the above groups, and recent immigrants from Haiti. The epidemiologic findings supported those who contended that an infectious agent was responsible for the severe immunosuppression common to the sufferers of AIDS. First, the outbreak of AIDS was clearly a new phenomenon, whether judged by clinicians who were seeing this severe syndrome in otherwise healthy people or measured by the dramatic increase in the requests for pentamidine, a drug used for the treatment of pneumocystis pneumonia and only available through CDC. Second, the disease was geographically localized, occurring primarily on the East and West coasts (and apparently spreading inland). Third, many of the early patients in Los Angeles and New York had had sexual contact.[1] Last, the groups involved, although socially very disparate, were, at least to epidemiologists, reminiscent of groups associated with other diseases.

When trying to assemble the pieces of a new disease puzzle, epidemiologists try to fit the disease's description into patterns of known diseases. These patterns often fit into different categories depending on the mechanism of transmission between people. This categorization can be extremely helpful to the laboratory investigator who is trying to find the causative agent. The causative agents of some diseases (e.g., polio and hepatitis A) are transmitted in feces and are spread in fecally contaminated environments. Others (e.g., measles and the common cold) are spread via contact with secretions from the upper respiratory tract. Still others (e.g., malaria and yellow fever) are transmitted via the bite of insects. None of these modes of transmission joined the disparate groups who had AIDS.

But another group of diseases did. These diseases, represented by hepatitis B, are spread by close, especially sexual, contact and are also spread via blood.[2] The virus that causes hepatitis B is primarily a blood-borne virus and exits infected persons via blood, serum, or semen. It is thus a relatively difficult virus to transmit, and the groups infected by it are rather limited. It is spread between homosexual contacts, heterosexual contacts, intravenous drug users who share needles, children and adults of the developing world, patients and health care workers, and infected mothers and their infants. With the exception of health care workers, the groups with AIDS are remarkably similar to those with hepatitis B virus infection.

The hepatitis B virus model also helped explain how such an outbreak might occur. Generally, blood-borne diseases do not spread easily between people (unless they involve mosquitoes or other insects in their transmission cycles). Thus, outbreaks of such diseases are rare. An "amplifier" of transmission would have to be present to augment the otherwise slow spread. The first outbreak of Ebola virus—the aggressive agent of African hemorrhagic fever—was a perfect example. I was a member of the 1976 World Health Organization team that rushed to the southwestern corner of Sudan when this disease had consumed several hundred people in short order. We suspect, but have never proven, that this virus hides in some animal and occasionally infects humans. Once in humans, this extremely dangerous blood-borne virus spreads only to extremely close contacts of victims. Thus, without an amplifier, the disease will burn itself out. In Sudan, there appeared to be two amplifiers. The first was a highly sexually active group in Nzara, the town where it started. And the second was modern medicine—a nurse training hospital in nearby Maridi where one of the initial patients was transferred. The close attention these nursing students paid to their patients cost half of them their lives and allowed a rapid expansion of the outbreak.[3]

The amplifier of the outbreak of AIDS appears to be the homosexual community—specifically those men who have sex with many other men in bathhouse-type settings. Homosexual activity is probably as old as mankind, but commercialized homosexual sex is a new phenomenon and is primarily concentrated in the large coastal cities that reported AIDS. These commercial establishments allow easy access to sexual partners. Thus, many men can have sex with men who in turn have had sex with many other men. This is an ideal setting for disease transmission, and the results of an introduction of a new infectious agent into this community would have predictable effects.

Where did this hypothetical agent come from? It could be either a radical modification of a known United States agent or a newly introduced one. The recent reports of European cases of an AIDS-like disease in persons from Africa[4] plus the American and European AIDS connection with Haiti lead one to speculate that this is an infection of Africans that has spread to the Caribbean and to the United States. Could it have been introduced purposely as some biological attack? There is certainly no evidence of this.

Although these speculations do not guarantee that AIDS is caused by a newly imported infectious agent that circulates in blood, many of the searches for a cause of AIDS have been directed toward proving or disproving this theory.

Before launching into what has been found or what has not been found regarding the cause of AIDS, I will review the methods and approaches that have been used to search out that cause.

Much like rescue teams looking for a lost hiker in a deep forest, laboratory teams look for both indirect evidence of presence—a footprint—and direct evidence—the hiker. They search likely areas for visible signs that might lead them to the cause. As a search helicopter first looks for large, easily visible signs, perhaps a tent or a puff of campfire smoke, the standard light microscope is used to search for some large visible change that might be unique. Some infectious agents themselves are visible under the miscroscope; other smaller organisms, such as viruses, are not. But some small viruses, because of the large numbers of virus particles present or because of a response of the infected host, produce unique structures that can be easily seen with standard light microscopes. An example of this is yellow fever virus, which, although far too small to be seen with the standard microscope, produces large virus "factories" that are visible in cells. These factories, called councilman bodies, were seen years before the discovery of the cause of yellow fever and are still helpful in making the diagnosis.

If the search at a distance is fruitless, then a closer look is required; for this the electron microscope is used. Yet, as in the search for the lost hiker, if one begins to look for footprints, one must limit the area of search because it is impossible to cover much area with small-object searching. Moreover, unless the concentration of markers is high (like finding footprints by chance at an abandoned campsite) the random chance of seeing a causative agent is extremely low. As a matter of fact, an electron microscope will not allow the viewer to see virus particles unless the concentration exceeds 1 million per milliliter (33,000 per drop). Thus, direct visualization of viruses, even in known infected tissues, is often difficult.

Yet, even when a causative agent is not visible, proof of infection can often be found. This proof often uses some system that increases the chance of discovery of the agent, like a test that detects structural parts of the agent or antibodies against the agent produced by the host. Antibodies are immunoglobulin proteins that are produced by animals when something foreign is discovered by their ever-vigilant immune system. These are highly specific and are produced in large amounts. Thus, they can be used as markers of a previous or ongoing infection.

Direct agent isolation is another and probably the ideal way to detect an infection. Most bacteria can be grown in the laboratory on special media with certain nutrients. They generally do not require living cells to grow. Viruses, on the other hand, do require living cells to replicate. They are extremely simple and grow by using constituents within living cells. Cells can be grown in the laboratory and inoculation with viruses can cause infection of the cells. However, there are several problems regarding virus isolation in cell culture that are especially pertinent with regard to AIDS.

The first problem is cell susceptibility to virus infection. Despite having several hundred cell lines from which to choose, many viruses grow only in one or a few lines and some do not grow at all. Secondly, some viruses grow in cell culture, but detecting their growth in these cells is difficult. Classic cell culture virology relies upon the destruction of cells to detect virus replication. Yet, we now know that some viruses can replicate in cells without destroying them. For these there is no easy endpoint such as cell death by which to judge if something is growing. One must rely on more elaborate detection methods through which, by some specific tool, one can "see" a virus. Some specific substances, such as antibody or nucleic acids, will identify viruses even if the cells remain alive. The problem here is that such methods can be developed only if we know what we are looking for. That is, if we are looking for a known virus we can vaccinate a guinea pig, for example, with pure virus. The guinea pig will produce antibody to that virus. Then serum from the guinea pig that contains the antibody can be "tagged" with something easily detectable—usually a radioisotope, whose activity is detectable by a counter, either an enzyme whose reactive product changes the color of the medium, or a pigment that will fluoresce when exposed to ultraviolet light (black light).

Obviously, though, if we don't know what virus we are searching for and we are thus unable to raise antibodies in guinea pigs, it is difficult to use these methods. With AIDS we are looking for a possible new virus. If the AIDS "agent" does not kill cell cultures, then how will we know it is there? Electron microscopes can be used, but again the virus must be in high concentrations to be detectable. Other techniques, such as those that use a tagged antibody, cannot be used because we do not know what antibody to use. In short, we would be looking for something that might or might not be there using techniques that might or might not work.

It would help to know that a transmissible agent did indeed cause AIDS. Since we would not and cannot use humans to establish this proof, we turn to animals. If we could produce AIDS in an animal then not only would we know that a transmissible agent causes the disease, but we could do multiple experiments to gain an understanding of the disease's course, transmission, and prevention. But, as in choosing the proper cell lines for cell culture inoculation, we must choose the proper animal. As with cells, viruses can be very restrictive regarding which animals they will infect. Ideally, an easily available, inexpensive animal, such as a mouse, would be susceptible. Then many experiments could be done at minimal cost. At the other extreme are nonhuman primates (monkeys and apes). If this "agent" is highly host-specific and will infect only primates, then the problem is greater. These animals are rare and expensive and require special and costly handling.

Recently an AIDS-like disease in monkeys was reported by two primate centers (one near Boston, Massachusetts, and one in Davis, California). In both of these centers, monkeys have been dying from diseases similar to that seen in AIDS patients, and the disease appears to be transmissible. Unfortunately, we seem to be as far from determining the cause of this disease as we are for AIDS. Whether it will be helpful as an animal model remains to be seen.

But even if we can find a susceptible animal for AIDS, how will we detect infection and how long will it take? If a disease similar to human AIDS develops in the animal or if similar alterations in cells of the immune system develop, then we can detect "infection." If not, we have no other marker at this stage. And even if AIDS does develop in an animal, it could take months to years—if it follows what appears to be the case in humans. Such long latent periods would obviously slow our pursuit of knowledge considerably.

So what has happened over the past years and what do we know regarding AIDS? Here I will focus on the efforts of CDC simply because I am most familiar with it, but many other institutions have put great effort into searching for the cause of AIDS. Those with which I am familiar I will mention, but my exclusion of others is a sign of my ignorance and is not meant to underestimate the efforts of others.

Mounting a massive effort to find the cause of AIDS, or for that matter the cause of any new disease, requires considerable resources—small maybe in terms of resources mobilized for military pursuits, but large in terms of budgets like CDC's. Indeed, the AIDS epidemic began at a time of constricting government budgets. As additional CDC funds were not available, the mobilization of staff and other resources for AIDS meant sacrificing other important disease control programs. Other government and non-government institutions have also devoted resources to these efforts as other research institutions have been willing and have made substantial commitments despite limited funds.

CDC's relationship nationally with local medical and public health facilities provides it with great access to information and specimens from patients. Also, it is traditionally CDC's role to search for new agents in these situations, be it AIDS, Legionnaires' disease, or toxic shock syndrome. For these reasons, CDC is expected to continue to play a major role in the continuing search for an etiologic agent.

The pursuit of an infectious agent for AIDS has been hampered by a disbelief that AIDS was (is) an infectious disease. Only in the past year has the infectious nature of this disease become acceptable within the scientific community. At a Public Health Service (Centers for Disease Control, National Institutes of Health, and the Food and Drug Administration) meeting on AIDS in March 1982, most support and interest centered around two possible causes: amyl and butyl nitrite inhalants ("poppers"), drugs used frequently by homosexual men, and sperm as an immunosuppressive substance. At that meeting, the epidemiologic similarities of AIDS and hepatitis B virus infection of humans and the virologic-mechanistic similarities of AIDS to feline leukemia virus infection of cats was discussed. The group was not yet ready to enthusiastically accept AIDS as an infectious disease. However, for those such as Dr. Curran, director of the CDC effort, knowledgeable about venereal diseases of homosexual men, there was a close parallel between AIDS and several diseases transmitted through sexual contact.

But the search has not been entirely limited to infectious agents. Groups at the National Institutes of Health (NIH) continued their work on the immune effects of sperm, and groups at CDC's National Institute for Occupational Safety and Health began animal experiments on the immunologic effects of amyl and butyl nitrite.

Most of the initial infectious disease–directed investigations centered around standard pathologic examination and attempts at agent isolation and identification via serologic antibody markers. These studies involved not just CDC staff; extensive work was done by the laboratories of the hospitals, primarily in New York, Los Angeles, and San Francisco, where scores of these patients began dying. Although not definitive regarding the cause of AIDS, the pathologic examinations of pre- and postmortem specimens from patients was impressive. The uniqueness and extent of the infections these patients exhibited was striking. The infections that killed them were caused by organisms that were common yet seldom caused disease. The main offenders were *Pneumocystis carinii,* a protozoal parasite, *Mycobacterium avium,* a bacterium, and cytomegalovirus (CMV), a virus. Not only is disease rarely seen with these infections, but the extent of disease and the lack of defensive response of the patients has been most remarkable.

The question remained: What was the underlying condition that allowed these otherwise benign infections to run rampant? CDC's laboratories have performed thousands of laboratory tests and the answer is still not in. What has been found is that infections of all types are common in these patients, especially the homosexual men. Almost all have shown evidence of infection with Epstein-Barr (EB) virus, the cause of mononucleosis, CMV, herpesvirus I and II, hepatitis B virus, and syphilis. In addition, infections with many other organisms are common. But from experience, we know or would expect that many infections would be common in people with multiple sexual partners, in users of intravenous drugs, and in people from developing countries. To determine if there is any unique infection in AIDS patients, comparative testing for infectious agents has been done on specimens from AIDS patients as well as non-AIDS-afflicted members of the same communities.

Jaffe and his co-workers at CDC collected blood and epidemiologic information from AIDS patients and healthy homosexual men of the same age in the same cities as patients. There were a few differences in the laboratory results from these comparative groups (see Table 1). First, although the same proportions of individuals from patient and comparative groups (called "controls") were infected by the agents tested, the AIDS patients had higher levels of antibody to several of the viruses tested (EB virus and CMV). Because CMV is known to cause suppression of the immune system after infection, special attention has been given to it. All homosexual patients (and almost all homosexual controls) have had antibody to CMV and have thus been infected at some time in the past. Only two AIDS patients tested to date have not had CMV antibodies. In addition, the concentration of CMV antibodies has been higher in AIDS patients than in controls. As for attempts to isolate a causative agent in cell culture, CMV has been the most common virus identified. If one does repeat virus cultures on AIDS patients on urine and other body fluids, CMV can be found in many if not all. But could CMV be the cause?

Dr. Drew and his co-workers in San Francisco showed several years ago that virtually all homosexual men are infected with CMV

Table 1

Antibody Testing to Various Infectious Agents
Comparison of Homosexual AIDS Patients and Homosexual Controls
from the Same Cities*

Agent	Percent Positive Patients (50)	Percent Positive Controls (117)
Cytomegalovirus	100	97–100
Epstein-Barr virus	100	100
Herpes simplex I	100	95–97
Herpes simplex II	98	90–97
Varicella zoster virus	76	91–100
Respiratory syncytial virus	68	71–94
Adenovirus	92	91–100
Chlamydia	51	67–68
Hepatitis B virus	94	85–92
Hepatitis A virus	86	54–63
Toxoplasma gondii	33	37–49
Entameba histolytica	6	0–7
Candida albicans	15	30–37
Syphilis	70	30–41

*Rogers, et al., *Annals of Internal Medicine*, 1983.

soon after they begin promiscuous sexual activity. But CMV causes its initial infection and then stays dormant indefinitely in body cells. Periodically, though, it reemerges from its latent state. This reactivation is known to be common when the infected person's immune system becomes less alert—for example, after cancer or chemotherapy. Dr. Drew asks then, is CMV a driver or a passenger in AIDS? Is it only another opportunist coming forth because of alteration in the immune system due to another agent or does it indeed cause AIDS? To help answer the question, Dr. Cabradilla at CDC studied different examples of CMV grown from different patients. He hypothesized that if CMV is the cause of this new disease, then a new CMV, unique from others, should be present in all cases. By examining the DNA of different isolates he found that they were indeed different. Although not completely established, it appears that CMV is a passenger in this disease. As a passenger it may be important, however, and further investigations are necessary.

What of other viruses? Besides a few adenovirus isolates, nothing has been striking. Investigators at CDC and elsewhere have looked extensively at many tissues from patients. In a collaborative study with Dr. Safai and his co-workers at Memorial Sloan-Kettering Hospital in New York and other collaborators in several cities, CDC investigators have intensively examined multiple tissues from several groups of patients. Nothing definite has been found.

Because of disease in hemophilia patients, Dr. Evatt and his group at CDC have looked extensively at concentrated Factor VIII material—the plasma-derived clotting factor that is used to counteract bleeding. Some passing views of particles that look like viruses have been seen by Dr. Palmer but nothing appears definite. The same group, together with Dr. Ewing, has used the electron microscope to search the tissues of patients. Again some interesting structures have been seen, but their exact meaning remains to be determined.

At the time of the early reports of AIDS, discussion began regarding the risk of AIDS for hospital and laboratory personnel who cared for patients or undertook AIDS research. CDC published recommendations regarding hospital isolation procedures in its *Morbidity and Mortality Weekly Reports*. The issue of safety for laboratory workers for AIDS really came to a head during the spring and summer of 1981. Much of the discussion centered around animal handlers who would take care of primates that had been injected with potentially infectious material. A review of laboratory practices at CDC at this time showed wide variations in precautions. Some of the busiest sections, especially those not directly involved with infectious agents, were dealing extremely casually with specimens. Others were quite careful. Dr. Feorino in Atlanta had been injecting laboratory mice for several months at that time, and he was indeed cautious. He limited his work to one safety room, and only he was allowed to do the injections.

But primates are somewhat different. They are smart and can be aggressive. The combination can be hazardous, as they can throw feces and actually connive to bite or scratch their handlers. The experience of CDC's primate handlers was extensive, and plans were made to ensure their safety and the safety of their immediate community contacts. Isolation suits were designed for the handlers, and rooms were modified so that the marmosets could be housed in their own safety structure and everything leaving their room could be disinfected or autoclaved. In August 1982, the first inoculations were made. Subsequently, chimpanzees in Atlanta were inoculated and Drs. Purcell and Sever and their co-workers at the National Institutes of Health inoculated several species of primates. Although these experiments have proceeded for several months in the longest case, no signs of disease have yet developed. However, if the evidence from the disease in humans is correct, the latent period could be as long as a year or two.

In summary, after over a year of pursuit, nothing definite has been observed despite considerable effort. Indeed, the interest in this disease among the scientific community is intense, and many researchers, in the face of inadequate funding, have pinched and squeezed to do something. A year might seem like a long time, but many of us felt early in the investigation that if the cause were not found immediately, it would take considerable time. It is evident now that it will not be easy. The cause does not appear to be a known, well-characterized infectious agent. Thus, the search is being widened. The past year, although somewhat frustrating, has not been without excitement. Periodically, bits and pieces come forth. They are not always true leads, but they nonetheless heighten the excitement. The current excitement comes from the laboratories of Dr. Essex at Harvard and Dr. Gallo at NIH. They, in collaboration with CDC, have produced some very interesting data regarding human T cell leukemia virus—a cancer-producing virus that Dr. Gallo discovered a few years ago. By a variety of techniques, these investigations have uncovered signs that this virus, which is known to produce clusters of leukemia in some parts of the world, commonly infects groups at risk of developing AIDS. Like other leads, this one has to be pursued to sort out the driver versus passenger problem that was mentioned regarding cyto-megalovirus.

So the exciting work continues. Hampered only by the lack of money, scientists from around the country and around the world are pressing nature to tell us how and why AIDS has caused such misery and death among our people.

Part V

The Future

The scope and complexity of the current AIDS epidemic outlined in this book clearly demands an active involvement by the federal government in the search for a solution to the crisis. As the disease spreads across our nation, and affects more and more communities, it becomes increasingly obvious that no local authority has the resources required to investigate, treat, or prevent the spread of AIDS.

We are fortunate to conclude this book with two thoughtful chapters by men who are in positions to fashion a national response. Dr. Donald Fredrickson is widely respected as the dean of American research, having served for many years as the Director of the National Institutes of Health. Before assuming his present foundation post he was also Scholar-in-Residence at the Institute of Medicine.

The political response—or lack thereof—to the AIDS epidemic is considered by Congressman Theodore Weiss, chairman of the House of Representatives oversight committee concerned with intergovernmental relations and human service appropriations. He calls for immediate federal action, and echoes the plea made by Cardinal Cooke at the beginning of this book—and reemphasized by every contributor—that both public and private health forces combine their strengths till the AIDS epidemic has been conquered and this dread disease is but another memory in the history of medicine.

12

Where Do We Go from Here?

Donald S. Fredrickson, M.D.

One by one the experts have come to tell us what they know about this new calamity, and by aligning the fragments differently we can catch various views of its dimensions. They are frightening. It is now only a few years since the first victims appeared. They were of a singular culture, promiscuous individuals having homosexual contacts with numerous and often anonymous untraceable persons. Mysteriously, they became the helpless prey of opportunistic infections and rare cancers, their resistance having been totally stripped away. The circle of the involved has now widened to include other cultures and lifestyles. The frequency of case reports is rising and so far nothing has proved effective in saving the lives of the stricken. They all have one common denominator. The helper T cell lymphocytes, which are the facilitators of the body's immunological defenses, have disappeared. The cause of this acquired immune deficiency syndrome (AIDS) now appears to be transmissible through sexual contact or exposure to contaminated blood and blood products. Although the epidemic movement of this pestilence is tightly restricted at present, we must consider everyone as potentially vulnerable.

Where do we go from here?

There is only one answer. We must find the cause and determine the modes of cure and prevention. And we will.

Some members of the communities most affected will undoubtedly view this answer as rhetoric. They will also consider the progress in combating this disease to be pitifully slow and blame traditional attitudes for blunting the attention their imminent danger requires.

Let me try to put these concerns in perspective. An epidemic signifies an intensified struggle for adaptation between man and some other species of life. The history of such calamities adds up to a balance in favor of man. We have reason to be cautiously optimistic.

Let's make some comparisons between the present situation and what we find in history. Thucydides' account of the plague in Athens in the time of Pericles is matter-of-fact and heartless.[1] But he does remind us of the difference between the state of ignorance then and the base of knowledge from which today's attack is being launched. In the fourteenth century, half of Europe died of the Black Death without the comfort of a hundredth of the bibliography about AIDS that is growing daily.[2] The same can be said of the pandemic of Spanish influenza of 1918–1919, considered by its major historian to have "killed more humans than any other disease in a period of similar duration in the history of the world."[3]

The practical instruction from each such episode outweighs the literature. The influenza epidemic, for example, gave us invaluable native experience in how variation in a pathogen combined with a marked change in life-style can have such a devastating effect on a human population. Even a bacterium of ancient lineage can be bumped from its obscure niche into a flare of dangerous expression. Such was the recent lesson from Legionella.

The solution of the enigma of any new disease demands the application of some old epidemiological virtues. The recent story of Lyme arthritis[4] illustrates the dogged persistence of a few academic investigators in pursuing the trail of an elusive disease and the value of an open mind on the part of a microbiologist who just happened to remember a lesson from his distant past as a trainee. Kuru, pursued with the same kind of fervor and alertness in an obscure culture, gave the world understanding of a whole other kind of pathogen, with an incubation period redolent of what we know of AIDS.[5] In addition to the slow viruses, there is even more recent awareness of a double agent, consisting of a defective pathogen and a helper; the delta antigen, too, gives us something to think about in this new disease.[6] All of these examples illustrate the great strength inherent in the combination of the old-fashioned virtues of skepticism and dedication combined with effective use of the burgeoning new technology.

The origin of the knowledge base relevant to AIDS merits a little more elaboration because it bears on how forces are being mobilized for the present defense. One must keep in mind that no government officials could have ordered, or any body of experts have suggested, preparation for a then invisible disease and achieved anything like the massive armamentarium now assembled.

Forty years ago the understanding of the immune system did not even amount to a pale outline of the detailed knowledge that is now accumulating at a phenomenal rate. Even twenty years ago the distinctions between lymphocytes crucial to the understanding of this disease could never have been recognized. From the recent revolution in biology, still in full excitement, have flowed techniques for identifying and separating lymphocytes at rates of thousands per second, for growing cells in culture, for fusing them to make great amounts of monoclonal antibodies, for capturing and defining both antigens and antibodies, and for determining the modes of communication between the numerous populations of cells that harbor the defect in AIDS. Similarly, brilliant illumination has fallen upon genetic control of biological systems and the creation of new technologies for manipulating them. Thus the possibilities constantly expand for the modeling and testing of hypotheses about normal processes and their aberrations. Being basically the same stuff as genes (DNA) or their immediate transcriptions (RNA), viruses are much more comprehensible to us today. Several viral infections, most notably hepatitis, have to be considered closely in the study of AIDS. Likewise viruses associated with leukemias in animals and possibly man are of similar interest in the new disease. Countless other areas of research in cancer, in the transplantation of tissues, in preparation of blood products or of vaccines, are also immediately adjacent to AIDS in this constantly expanding universe of biological knowledge.

This is the fruit of a worldwide endeavor that recognizes no national boundaries. A very large portion of the activity has been generated by a wise and generous investment made in biomedical research by the American people through the federal government beginning about 1950. The same support was accompanied by development of a system for scientific inquiry in the nation's universities and teaching hospitals that is unparalleled in any other period of our history. The state of preparedness for the war on AIDS is partly a reflection of the design and philosophy of the Public Health Service, now under the Department of Health and Human Services. In the fight against AIDS, the Centers for Disease Control (CDC), the National Institutes of Health (NIH), and the Food and Drug Administration (FDA) have specific and complementary roles. CDC is the experienced sentinel whose persistent scanning for evidence of clustering of disease was the principal means leading to awareness of AIDS. This agency has also developed the principal field force of epidemiologists who track down the contacts, collect the samples, and sift the early clues. CDC's resources are complemented by the massive resources of NIH. This agency is conducting an important part of the AIDS investigation in its own laboratories and clinics. It is also through NIH that the largest share of university and medical center laboratories of the nation are supported by federal funds. The methods for disbursing these funds are based on peer review systems and mechanisms that should allay suspicions that all the attention is on diseases occurring in larger numbers or affecting populations with more political appeal than the 1,300-some sufferers from AIDS. Much of the knowledge detailed above and elsewhere in this symposium is derived from the ability of NIH to support fundamental research relevant to all diseases. Elsewhere I have called this capacity the Venetian principle of NIH.[7] On the surface of its organization one sees the prominent structures erected by anxiety over the "great diseases"—cancer, arthritis, heart disease, and so forth. But below the surface the foundation is freely miscible. Although cynics have observed that Venice is sinking, the water (basic knowledge) is rising!

Enough of praise of this system. What is it doing in the case of AIDS? I have recently had opportunity to examine the organization of the Department of Health and Human Services (DHHS) agencies in regard to AIDS and as directed by the Assistant Secretary for Health. The roles are clear and the coordination of activities are sensibly arranged. The quality of people and resources committed to AIDS research in New York City and nationwide is impressive. The quantity of support is difficult to appraise, but I will say something of this later.

This analysis is cursory and the injunction to stay calm is not an invitation to complacency. The ring has not been closed. AIDS still eludes capture and definition. The effort we are making to contain this serious danger is obviously not enough. Congressman Weiss, who follows me to this platform, has indicated that he may seek congressional hearings on the federal role in this catastrophe. I would commend attention to several of the relevant facts, which include a glaring deficiency or two in our armor and some still hidden weaknesses giving cause for concern.

First, AIDS will not be conquered soon without an intensive and complete gathering of the facts. In America we have been limping along with a chronic deficiency of epidemiologists. The kinds we miss the most include those gifted in the sleuthing of infectious diseases. The burden of tracking down the contacts and collecting the samples is a huge one. I cannot believe that the elite corps of the CDC and the legion of its alumni now working in the states is of sufficient numbers for the job to be done with dispatch.

Second, as strong and praiseworthy as is America's biomedical research effort, it has been contracting in size during the past several years. There are no sources of private funds sufficient to close the gap. I have earlier alluded to reasons why the full strengths of funds allotted to the solution of specific disease problems are likely to be underestimates. There is a danger, however, in depending too much on the strength of the general tide of incoming fundamental knowledge. Its application to particular problems requires specific addition of funds. Congressional mandates for dedication of resources to solve specific problems, without additional appropriations, drain people and monies from other tasks. I can say from deep personal knowledge that the budgets for both CDC and the National Institute for Allergy and Infectious Diseases have not been adjusted to the level of new needs and opportunities for research into infectious diseases in the last few years. Both agencies will undoubtedly require additional funds to sustain the proper attack on AIDS, in its present projection.

Finally, it is important for all of us to be aware that, in the current economic crisis, the federal government, and now many of the states, are turning their backs on meeting the costs of health care for many of the disadvantaged. This is placing unusual strain on many of the hospitals and academic teaching centers where the essential research on AIDS is being conducted. Any increase in patients with AIDS, whose needs for long-term tertiary care are overwhelming, means that supplementation is going to be absolutely necessary.

In a medical emergency as severe and scientifically challenging as AIDS, there is potential for chaos. Such cannot be avoided by paramilitary organization but by unusual self-discipline and cooperation among all concerned. The worst danger is that the steady flow of information be obstructed. Careful and complete reporting of all cases to a central location, properly the CDC in this instance, is but one aspect of the necessarily universal approach to such a disease puzzle. Many lives may hang on the care with which data, samples, experimental results, and ideas are shared unselfishly. Rivalry that leads to compartmentalization is bad for science and perhaps fatal for patients. It has been encouraging to learn at this symposium about the high degree of cooperation among the centers of research in New York City. Each month there is now a regular meeting attended by representatives of each center and representatives of the communities most affected, sponsored by the Department of Health. Such interaction in the metropolitan area having the highest number of cases in the world is certainly appropriate to the scale of this catastrophe.

Obviously, one of the most pressing needs is for a specific marker for the disease. Without it, approaches to the containment of AIDS are clumsy. There is the danger of abuses through too much zeal in restrictive practices. There is the alternate risk of equivocation. There has to be a continuous and conscientious search for the middle ground, a search in which the affected communities clearly need to participate. This is becoming particularly important now as the data seem to make it clear that AIDS is transmissible through blood or blood products. Dawson's call for recognition of the risks of infected blood elsewhere in this symposium strikes me as realistic. A failure to urge proper precautions upon handlers of blood and other materials from patients suspected to have AIDS is not excusable. Neither is the generation of suspicion or fear that is not based on adequate information. The official pronouncements and the coverage by the media require unusual sensitivity in the instance of this disease.

A final injunction is perhaps not necessary, yet in every way it is the most important. This new plague shares one aspect with all the old ones. People have a fear of the sufferers. It can lead to their rejection and a rationalizing away of responsibilities. In the instance of the hospital worker, nurse, and physician, no compromise with the age-old duties of our vocations is acceptable. It is only this thin mantle of professionalism that separates these callings from the trades. Likewise, objectivity, frankness, and mutual respect for privacy and individual difference must be at center stage. Moral judgments and parochial sociology must be relegated to the wings.

The present sufferers from AIDS are not on the fringes of society, but in the vanguard of civilization. The deadly force to which they have fallen may lie in wait for any of us or perhaps our succeeding generations. Patients whose disease we do not understand perform an essential service for mankind. They may give up their lives to point out areas of ignorance where common danger lies.

13

The Public Response

Theodore Weiss, U.S. Representative

I am pleased to join this distinguished group of physicians and scientists to address what may be the greatest health peril since polio. This symposium provides an important opportunity for experts to share information and insights with each other and with all those who play a vital role in the effort to battle Acquired Immune Deficiency Syndrome (AIDS) and to care for its victims.

Earlier chapters have explored the epidemiological, medical, and scientific aspects of what is fact and what is conjecture about AIDS. Needless to say, I approach this subject with a lay person's perspective; my role as a member of Congress involves the politics and policies that affect this country's response to health emergencies and its efforts to safeguard and promote public health and well-being.

Unfortunately, this responsibility usually translates into fragmented year-to-year, program-by-program, and budget line-by-budget line policymaking. It's rare that Congress has the time or the inclination to examine fully and act upon the complexities of health policy and health care in this country. Similarly, many medical professionals allocate most of their time and resources on a patient-by-patient, disease-by-disease, treatment-by-treatment basis. They, too, have little energy to devote to the many issues in health policy and delivery.

The AIDS crisis warrants more than a business-as-usual response from both government and the medical-scientific establishment. It demands immediate, exhaustive, and coordinated action to discover causes, treatments, and prevention of AIDS. It demands a concerted effort to educate the public with accurate medical information. And it demands a special sensitivity to the individuals and communities that have fallen victim to this catastrophic affliction. The human tragedy of this outbreak is deepened by the youth of the victims, the debilitating and costly nature of their illness, and the lack of any concrete information about its cause or cure.

It has become clear that the fight to discover a cure for AIDS is one of the most difficult struggles the medical-scientific community has ever faced, and perhaps will ever face. This is because what we are all battling is more than a disease epidemic. As you know, three-quarters of all victims are gay men. One cannot separate societal reticence to address the AIDS epidemic from the larger problem of resistance to basic civil rights protection for gays. In the past, disregard for their human rights has cost them job security, housing, adequate health care, and free self-expression. With the outbreak of AIDS, it is costing them their lives.

The national response from government, the medical community, the media, and the public at large has been less than zealous when compared to the reactions which followed outbreaks of toxic shock and Legionnaire's disease. And, although AIDS has taken twice as many lives as those two epidemics combined, the country has not been alerted, nor have our enormous resources been mobilized as quickly, as urgently, or as extensively as the situation warrants. For nearly two years, neither the government nor the medical community has accepted its leadership fully or devoted sufficient expertise in fighting this insidious epidemic. The achievements of the gay community in fighting this health emergency have laid the groundwork from which a more comprehensive effort must be built.

This is no time to indulge in irrational prejudices. We must focus on what really needs to be done: extinguishing the epidemic, preventing and curing the disorder, and caring for the afflicted.

In recent months, as AIDS cases and deaths have escalated at an alarming rate, a corresponding collective response to the epidemic has begun to develop. It is clear that as a society, we can no longer afford a haphazard response to this public health crisis. We are beginning to recognize that the tragedy now striking gay men, Haitians, hemophiliacs, and drug users is, in fact, a national tragedy.

Any course of future action must be developed and executed in a cooperative manner involving victims, health providers, government, concerned citizens, and organizations. Unilateral decision-making and exclusionary dialogue have no place in this crisis, particularly given the widespread misinformation about and discrimination against many of those devastated by the outbreak.

All of us who share a commitment to an aggressive response have much work to do.

First, Congress and the Administration must act quickly to allocate additional resources to maintain and expand public health surveillance and epidemiological research on AIDS. Thus far, the Centers for Disease Control (CDC), in conjunction with local and state health departments, has been stretched to the limit in its capacity to cope with AIDS. CDC desperately needs resources to expand surveillance work with health departments in cities hard hit by the AIDS epidemic. New York is the only city thus far to have such an arrangement with the agency. In addition, CDC needs funding to conduct extensive epidemiological investigations and long-term follow-up studies on all emerging risk groups. Patients are dying before CDC investigators are able to collect vital histories and information about possible patterns of AIDS transmission. Finally, CDC needs financial support for the laboratory work essential to isolate the cause of AIDS. Public support, particularly from the medical community, is essential to force Congress and the Administration to rethink budget priorities that damage public health and impede efforts to fight AIDS.

A second concern is the slow response of the National Institutes of Health (NIH) to initiate biomedical research on AIDS. The National Cancer Institute's first "request for application" (RFA) for research on AIDS was issued a year and a half into the outbreak. Its estimated 1983 expenditures for AIDS-related research amount to a mere one-fifth of one percent of the entire $4 billion NIH budget, or approximately $8 million. Dozens of scientists across the country are clamoring to do research on AIDS and waiting for NIH to allocate additional money. While NIH deliberates over how to spend this embarrassingly small allocation, vital research is put on hold, and individuals continue to die.

Third, physicians and medical associations must assume greater responsibility for educating all health providers on the most up-to-date information available on AIDS. Through continuing education, in-service training, research symposia, and medical journals, medical professionals can be better prepared to properly screen, diagnose, and care for AIDS patients.

AIDS is spreading fast. This makes it especially critical for the medical community to constantly disseminate new information about the epidemic. Networks for medical referrals and consultations must be expanded and promoted. And it is very important that the medical community strive for a greater understanding of and sensitivity to the needs of the various populations victimized by the disease.

I also believe that this public health crisis warrants an outpouring of psychological and social support for afflicted patients and communities. The demand for services in cities such as New York, Los Angeles, San Francisco, Houston, and Washington, D.C., is staggering. Needed services cover a broad spectrum: individual and group therapy, legal assistance, home care, hospice care, medical referrals, crisis interven-tion, and guidance through the maze of public assistance, health, and disability programs. Compassion has guided tireless efforts to help AIDS victims as well as their friends and families cope with the reality of this life-threatening disorder. In many instances, patients need additional support to deal with the feelings of isolation and loss that result from disruptions in their jobs, personal lives, and social networks.

Even with these support systems, the needs are growing faster than available financial and human resources. Additional volunteers, particularly those with professional expertise, are needed to lend a hand. Money, supplies, and even space must be contributed gener-ously by well-established social and human service organizations as well as by government agencies. AIDS causes widespread human tragedy—it demands the most active and human response our society can give.

It has been estimated that treatment for the first 300 AIDS cases cost a total of $18 million, or $60,000 per case on average. The caseload has quadrupled and continues to grow at an alarming rate. Most AIDS patients are unable to afford such astronomical costs for medical care. Many have lost insurance coverage because their debilitating condition leaves them unable to work. Many have exhausted their insurance coverage because of the catastrophic nature of the illness. Most do not qualify for public assistance. The cost of medical treatment is so exorbitant that some patients may be forced to choose between their homes and their health care. I believe that both government and the medical community must launch a joint effort to ensure that victims of this epidemic do not want for medical care because they lack sufficient resources.

I feel that the active response of the gay community, coupled with the slowly building sense of urgency demonstrated in the medical field, fuels hope for a positive resolution to the AIDS crisis. But as we crawl toward a solution, lives continue to be lost. The air of national emergency and collective sensitivity that put Legionnaires' disease on the front pages of newspapers across the country and kept it there until the problem was solved is still lacking.

Research on AIDS may provide us with a better working knowledge of the immune system, infectious diseases, and cancer. But until the entire nation is alerted that AIDS is a serious public health danger, capable of enveloping huge numbers of people at any time, the reality exists that our efforts may prove to be too little, and too late. A caring and responsible society must not allow that to happen.

Notes and Sources

Note to the Reader

Because of the urgent need to get this book to medical practitioners and the general public as quickly as possible, there was not enough time to make consistent the diverse reference systems used by each writer, for which anomaly we apologize.

—The Publisher

Chapter 3. The Haitian Connection

SOURCES

Brunet, J. B., and the Study Group on the Epidemiology of AIDS in France. "Acquired immunodeficiency in France." *Lancet* 1 (1983): 700–701.

Liautaud, B., Laroche, C., Duvivier, J., et al. "Le sarcome de Kopsi (maladie de Kaposi) est-il frequent en Haiti?" Presented in April 1982 at the 18th Congrès des Médecins Francophones de l'Hemisphère Americain, Port-au-Prince, Haiti.

Pitchenik, A. E., Fischl, M., Dickinson, G. M., et al. "Acquired immune deficiency in Haitians: opportunistic infections in previously healthy Haitian immigrants." *N. Engl. J. Med.* 308 (1983): 125.

Colton, R. M., and Spira, T. J. "Opportunistic infections and Kaposi's sarcoma." *Ann. Intern. Med.* 98 (1983): 277.

Chapter 4: Immunologic Aberrations: The AIDS Defect

SOURCES

Editorial: "Immunocompromised Homosexuals." *Lancet* 2 (1981):1325–1329.

Autran, Br., Gorin, I., Leibowitch, M., et al. "AIDS in a Haitian woman with cardiac Kaposi's sarcoma and Whipple's disease." *Lancet* 1 (1983):767–768.

Babb, R. R.. "Sexually transmitted infections in homosexual men." *Postgrad. Medicine* 65 (1979):215–218.

Bachman, D. M., Rodrigues, M. M., Chu, F. C., et al. "Culture-proven cytomegalovirus retinitis in a homosexual man with the acquired immunodeficiency syndrome." *Amer. Acad. of Ophthalmology* 89 (1982):797–804.

Biggar, R. J., Melbye, M., Ebbesen, P., et al. "Immunsuppressionssyndromet hos homoseksuelle maend." *Ugeskr Laeger* 144 (1982):777–780.

Boldogh, I., Beth, E., Huang, E.-S., et al. "Kaposi's sarcoma. IV. Detection of CMV DNA, CMV RNA and CMNA in tumor biopsies." *Int. J. Cancer* 28 (1981):469–474.

Brennan, R. O. and Durack, D. T. "Gay compromise syndrome." *Lancet* 2 (1981): 1338–1339.

Brunet, J. B., and the Study Group on the Epidemiology of AIDS in France. "Acquired immunodeficiency syndrome in France." *Lancet* 1 (1983):700–701.

Clumeck, N., Mascart-Lemone, F., de Maubeuge, J., et al. "Acquired immune deficiency syndrome in black Africans." *Lancet* 1 (1983):642.

Cunningham-Rundles, S., Michelis, M. A., and Masur, H. "Serum suppression of lymphocyte activation in vitro in acquired immunodeficiency disease." *J. Clin. Immunol.* 3 (1983): 156–165.

Davis, K. C., Hayward, A., Ozturk, G., et al. "Lymphocyte transfusion in case of acquired immunodeficiency syndrome." *Lancet* 1 (1983): 599–600.

Deodhar, S. D., Kuklinga, A. G., Vidt, D. G., et al. "Development of reticulum-cell sarcoma at the site of antilymphocyte globulin injection in a patient with renal transplant." *N. Engl. J. Med.* 280 (1969): 1104–1106.

Desforges, J. F. "AIDS and preventive treatment in hemophilia." *N. Engl. J. Med.* 308 (1983): 94–95.

DeWys, W. D., Curran, J., Henle, W., et al. "Workshop on Kaposi's sarcoma: meeting report." *Cancer Treatment Repts.* 66 (1982): 1387–1390.

Drew, W. L., Mintz, L., Miner, R. C., et al. "Prevalence of cytomegalovirus infection in homosexual men." *J. Infect. Dis.* 143 (1981): 188–192.

Ellis, W. R., Coleman, J. C., Fluker, J. L., et al. "Liver disease among homosexual males." *Lancet* (April 28, 1979): 903–905.

Fauci, A. S. "The syndrome of Kaposi's sarcoma and opportunistic infections: an epidemiologically restricted disorder of immunoregulation." *Ann. Intern. Med.* 96 (1982): 777–779.

Felman, Y. M. and Nikitas, J. A. "Sexually transmitted viral hepatitis." *N.Y. State J. Med.* (January 1980): 64–66.

Fluker, J. L. "A 10-year study of homosexually transmitted infection." *Brit. J. Vener. Dis.* 52 (1976): 155–160.

Follansbee, S. E., Busch, D. F., Wofsy, C. B., et al. "An outbreak of *Pneumocystis carinii* pneumonia in homosexual men." *Ann. Intern. Med.* 96 (1982): 705–713.

Francioli, P., Vogt, M., Schadelin, J., et al. "Syndrome de déficience immunitaire acquisé, infections opportunistes et homosexualité. Présentation de 3 cas observés en Suisse." *Schweiz. med. Wschr.* 112 (1982): 1682–1687.

Francioli, P. and Clement, F. "Beta$_2$-microglobulin and immunodeficiency in a homosexual man." *N. Engl. J. Med.* 307 (1982): 1402–1403.

Friedman, S. M., Felman, Y. M., Rothenberg, R., et al. "Follow-up on Kaposi's sarcoma and *Pneumocystis* pneumonia." *Morbidity and Mortality Weekly Report* 30 (1981): 409–410.

Friedman, S. M., Laubenstein, L., Marmor, M., et al. "Kaposi's sarcoma and *Pneumocystis* pneumonia among homosexual men—New York City and California." *Morbidity and Mortality Weekly Report* 30 (1981): 305–308.

Friedman-Kein, A. E., Laubenstein, L. J., Rubinstein, P., et al. "Disseminated Kaposi's sarcoma in homosexual men." *Ann. Intern. Med.* 96 (1982): 693–700.

Frizzera, G., Rosai, J., Dehner, L. P., et al. "Lymphoreticular disorders in primary immunodeficiencies: new findings based on an up-to-date histologic classification of 35 cases." *Cancer* 46 (1980): 692–699.

Gardiner, R. "Incidence of nodular lymphoid hyperplasia in homosexual men." *AJR* 138 (1982): 593.

Gilkey, F. W. "Opportunistic infections and Kaposi's sarcoma in homosexual men" (Letter to editor). *N. Engl. J. Med.* 306 (1982): 934.

Giraldo, G., Beth, E., and Haguenau, F. "Herpes-type virus particles in tissue culture of Kaposi's sarcoma from different geographic regions." *J. Natl. Cancer Inst.* 49 (1972): 1509–1526.

Giraldo, G., Beth, E., Coeur, P., et al. "Kaposi's sarcoma: a new model in the search for viruses associated with human malignancies." *J. Natl. Cancer Inst.* 49 (1972): 1495–1507.

Giraldo, G., Beth, E., and Huang, E.-S. "Kaposi's sarcoma and its relationship to cytomegalovirus (CMV) III. CMV DNA and CMV early antigens in Kaposi's sarcoma." *Int. J. Cancer* 26 (1980): 23–39.

Godwin, J. D., Ravin, C. E., and Roggli, V. L. "Fatal *Pneumocystis* pneumonia, cryptococcosis, and Kaposi's sarcoma in a homosexual man." *AJR* 138 (1982): 580–581.

Golden, J. "*Pneumocystis* lung disease in homosexual men." Medical Staff Conference, U. of CA, San Francisco School of Med., *West. J. Med.* 137 (1982): 400–407.

Gottlieb, M. S., Schroff, R., Schanker, H. M., et al. "*Pneumocystis carinii* pneumonia and mucosal candidiasis in previously healthy homosexual men." *N. Engl. J. Med.* 305 (1981): 1425–1431.

Greenberg, F. and Enlow, R. W. "Screening for risk of acquired immune-deficiency syndrome." *N. Engl. J. Med.* 307 (1982): 1521–1522.

Greene, J. B., Sidhu, G. S., Lewin, S., et al. "*Mycobacterium avium-intracellulare:* A cause of disseminated life-threatening infection in homosexuals and drug abusers." *Ann. Intern. Med.* 97 (1982): 539–546.

Groopman, J. E. and Gottlieb, M. S. "Kaposi's sarcoma: an oncologic looking glass." *Nature* 299 (1982): 103–104.

Guill, M. F. "Defects in cell-mediated immunity." *J. of MAG* 71 (1982): 607–609.

Gupta, S. and Safai, B. "Deficient autologous mixed lymphocyte reaction in Kaposi's sarcoma associated with deficiency of Leu-3+ responder T cells." *J. Clin. Invest.* 71 (1983): 296–300.

Gyorkey, F., Sinkovics, J. G., and Gyorkey, P. "Tubuloreticular structures in Kaposi's sarcoma." *Lancet* 2 (1982): 984–985.

Harwood, A. R., Osoba, D., Hofstader, S. L., et al. "Kaposi's sarcoma in recipients of renal transplants." *Am. J. Med.* 67 (1979): 759–765.

Hersh, E. M., Reuben, J. M., Rios, A., et al. "Elevated serum thymosin alpha-1 levels associated with evidence of immune dysregulation in male homosexuals with a history of infectious diseases or Kaposi's sarcoma." *N. Engl. J. Med.* 308 (1983): 45–46.

Holland, G. N., Gottlieb, M. S., Yee, R. D., et al. "Ocular disorders associated with a new severe acquired cellular immunodeficiency syndrome." *Am. J. Ophthalmology* 93

(1982): 393–402.

Johnson, R., Horwitz, D. N., and Frost, P. "Disseminated Kaposi's sarcoma in a homosexual man." *J. Am. Med. Assoc.* 247 (1982): 1739–1741.

Jorgensen, K. A., and Lawesson, S.-O. "Amyl nitrite and Kaposi's sarcoma in homosexual men." *N. Engl. J. Med.* 307 (1982): 893–894.

Koziner, B., Denny, T., Myskowski, P. L., et al. "Opportunistic infections and Kaposi's sarcoma in homosexual men" (Letter to the editor). *N. Engl. J. Med.* 306 (1982): 933–934.

Leggiadro, R. J., Winkelstein, J. A., and Hughes, W. T. "Prevalence of *Pneumocystis carinii* pneumonitis in severe combined immunodeficiency." *J. Ped.* 99 (1981): 96–98.

Levine, A. S. "The epidemic of acquired immune dysfunction in homosexual men and its sequelae-opportunistic infections, Kaposi's sarcoma, and other malignancies: an update and interpretation." *Cancer Treatment Repts.* 66 (1982): 1391–1395.

Lyon, M. F. and Loutit, J. F. "X-linked factor in acquired immunodeficiency syndrome?" *Lancet* 1 (1983): 768.

Macek, C. "Acquired immunodeficiency syndrome cause(s) still elusive." *J. Am. Med. Assoc.* 248 (1982): 1423–1431.

Masci, J. P., and Nicholas, P. "Precautions recommended in treating patients with AIDS." *N. Engl. J. Med.* 308 (1983): 156.

Masur, H., Michelis, M. A., and Wormser, G. P. "Acquired immune deficiency: the outbreak now extends to women." *Ann. Intern. Med.* 97 (1982): 533–539.

Masur, H., Michelis, M. A., Greene, J. B., et al. "An outbreak of community-acquired *Pneumocystis carinii* pneumonia: initial manifestation of cellular immune dysfunction." *N. Engl. J. Med.* 305 (1981): 1431–1438.

Masur, H., Michelis, M. A., Wormser, G. P., et al. "Opportunistic infection in previously healthy women. Initial manifestations of a community-acquired cellular immunodeficiency." *Ann. Intern. Med.* 97 (1982): 533–539.

McNutt, N. S., Fletcher, V., and Conant, M. A. "Early lesions of Kaposi's sarcoma in homosexual men. An ultrastructural comparison with other vascular proliferations in skin." *Am. J. Pathol.* 111 (1983): 62–77.

Mildvan, D., Mathur, U., Enlow, R. W., et al. "Persistent, generalized lymphadenopathy among homosexual males." *Morbidity and Mortality Weekly Report* 31 (1982): 249–251.

Mildvan, D., Mathur, U., Enlow, R. W., et al. "Opportunistic infections and immune deficiency in homosexual men." *Ann. Intern. Med.* 96 (1982): 700–704.

Miller, J. R., Barrett, R. E., Britton, C. B., et al. "Progressive multifocal leukoencephalopathy in a male homosexual with T-cell immune deficiency." *N. Engl. J. Med.* 307 (1982): 1436–1438.

Morris, L., Distenfeld, A., Amorosi, E., et al. "Autoimmune thrombocytopenic purpura in homosexual men." *Ann. Intern. Med.* 96 (1982): 714–717.

Myers, B. D., Kessler, E., Levi, J., Pick, A., Rosenfeld, J. B., and Tikvah, P. "Kaposi sarcoma in kidney transplant recipients." *Arch. Intern. Med.* 133 (1974): 307–311.

Myskowski, P. L., Romano, J. F., and Safai, B. "Kaposi's sarcoma in young homosexual men." *CUTIS* 29 (1982): 31–34.

Nahas, G. G. "Opportunistic infections and Kaposi's sarcoma in homosexual men" (Letter to the editor). *N. Engl. J. Med.* 306 (1982): 932.

Navarro, C. and Hagstrom, J. W. C. "Opportunistic infections and Kaposi's sarcoma in homosexual men" (Letter to the editor). *N. Engl. J. Med.* 306 (1982): 933.

Neumann, H. H. "Opportunistic infections and Kaposi's sarcoma in homosexual men"

(Letter to the editor). *N. Engl. J. Med.* 306 (1982): 935.

Neuwirth, J., Gutman, I., Hofeldt, A. J., et al. "Cytomegalovirus retinitis in a young homosexual male with acquired immunodeficiency." *Ophthalmology* 89 (1982): 805–808.

Nichols, P. W. "Opportunistic infections and Kaposi's sarcoma in homosexual men" (Letter to the editor). *N. Engl. J. Med.* 306 (1982): 934–935.

Oettle, A. G. "Geographical and racial differences in the frequency of Kaposi's sarcoma as evidence of environmental or genetic causes." *Acta Un. Int. Cancer* 18 (1962): 330–363.

Penn, I. "Kaposi's sarcoma in organ transplant recipients. Report of 20 cases." *Transplantation* 27 (1979): 8–11.

Penn, I., Halgrimson, C. G., and Starzl, T. E. "De Novo malignant tumors in organ transplant recipients." *Transpl. Proc.* III (1971): 773–778.

Ragni, M. V., Lewis, J. H., Spero, J. A., et al. "Acquired immunodeficiency syndrome in two haemophiliacs." *Lancet* 1 (1983): 213–214.

Rinaldo, Jr., C. R., Carney, W. P., Richter, B. S., et al. "Mechanisms of immunosuppression in cytomegaloviral mononucleosis." *J. Infect. Dis.* 141 (1980): 488–494.

Rothman, S. "Some clinical aspects of Kaposi's sarcoma in the European and North American population." *Acta Un. Int. Cancer* 18 (1962): 364–371.

Salmon, D., Landre, M.-F., Fraser, G. R., et al. "A familial aggregate of common variable immunodeficiency. Hodgkin disease and other malignancies in New-foundland—II. Genealogical analysis and conclusions regarding hereditary determinants." *Clin. & Invest. Med.* 2 (1980): 175–181.

Shearer, G. M. "Allogeneic leukocytes as a possible factor in induction of AIDS in homosexual men." *N. Engl. J. Med.* 308 (1983): 223–224.

Siegal, F. P. "Normal delayed-type skin reactions in early stages of acquired cellular immunodeficiency." *N. Engl. J. Med.* 307 (1982): 184.

Siegal, F. P., Lopez, C., Hammer, G. S., et al. "Severe acquired immunodeficiency in male homosexuals, manifested by chronic perianal ulcerative herpes simplex lesions." *N. Engl. J. Med.* 305 (1981): 1439–1444.

Siegel, J. H., Janis, R., Alper, J. C., et al. "Disseminated visceral Kaposi's sarcoma. Appearance after human renal homograft operation." *J. Am. Med. Assoc.* 207 (1969): 1493–1496.

Small, C. B., Klein, R. S., Friedland, G. H., et al. "Community-acquired opportunistic infections and defective cellular immunity in heterosexual drug abusers and homosexual men." *Am. J. Med.* 74 (1983): 433–441.

Snider, W. D., Simpson, D. M., Aronyk, K. E., et al. "Primary lymphoma of the nervous system associated with acquired immune-deficiency syndrome." *N. Engl. J. Med.* 308 (1983): 45.

Taff, M. L., Siegal, F. P., and Geller, S. A. "Outbreak of an acquired immunodeficiency syndrome associated with opportunistic infections and Kaposi's sarcoma in male homosexuals. An epidemic with forensic implications." *Am. J. Forensic Med. and Pathol.* 3 (1982): 259–264.

Thin, R. N. and Smith, D. M. "Some characteristics of homosexual men." *Brit. J. Vener. Dis.* 52 (1976): 161–164.

Urmacher, C., Myskowski, P., Ochoa, Jr., M., et al. "Outbreak of Kaposi's sarcoma with cytomegalovirus infection in young homosexual men." *Am. J. Med.* 72 (1982): 569–575.

Vanley, G. T., Huberman, R., and Lufkin, R. B. "Atypical *Pneumocystis carinii* pneumonia in homosexual men with unusual immunodeficiency." *Amer. J. Roent.* 138 (1982): 1037–1041.

Vieira, J., Frank, E., Spira, T. J., et al. "Acquired immune deficiency in Haitians. Opportunistic infections in previously healthy Haitian immigrants." *N. Engl. J. Med.* 308 (1983): 125–129.

Volberding, P., Conant, M. A., Stricker, R. B., et al. "Chemotherapy in advanced Kaposi's sarcoma. Implications for current cases in homosexual men." *Am. J. Med.* 74 (1983): 652–656.

Wood, R. W. "Opportunistic infections and Kaposi's sarcoma in homosexual men" (Letter to the editor). *N. Engl. J. of Med.* 306 (1982): 932–933.

Zakowski, P., Fligiel, S., Berlin, O. G. W., et al. "Disseminated *Mycobacterium avium-intracellulare* infection in homosexual men dying of acquired immunodeficiency." *J. Am. Med. Assoc.* 248 (1982): 2980–2982.

Zucker-Franklin, D. " 'Looking' for the cause of AIDS." *N. Engl. J. Med.* 308 (1983): 837–838.

Chapter 6. Bacterial and Mycotic Infections

NOTES

1. M. Poon, A. Landay, E. F. Prasthofer et al., "Acquired immunodeficiency syndrome with *Pneumocystis carinii* pneumonia and *Mycobacterium avium-intracellulare* infection in a previously healthy patient with classic hemophilia," *Ann. Intern. Med.* 98(1983): 287.

2. M. S. Gottlieb, R. Schroff, H. M. Schanker et al., "*Pneumocystis carinii* and mucosal candidiasis in previously healthy homosexual men: evidence of a new acquired cellular immunodeficiency," *N. Engl. J. Med.* 305 (1981): 1425.

   D. Mildvan, U. Mathur, R. W. Enlow et al., "Opportunistic infections and immune deficiency in homosexual men," *Ann. Intern. Med.* 96 (1982): 700.

   H. Masur, M. A. Michelis, J. B. Greene et al., "An outbreak of community-acquired *Pneumocystis carinii* pneumonia," *N. Engl. J. Med.* 305 (1981): 1431.

   H. Masur, M. A. Michelis, G. P. Wormer et al., "Opportunistic infections in previously healthy women," *Ann. Intern. Med.* 97 (1982): 533.

   F. P. Siegal, C. Lopez, G. S. Hammer et al., "Severe acquired immunodeficiency in male homosexuals manifested by chronic perianal ulcerative herpes simplex lesions," *N. Engl. J. Med.* 305 (1981): 1439.

   K. C. Davis, C. R. Horsburgh, U. Hasiba et al., "Acquired immunodeficiency syndrome in a patient with hemophilia," *Ann. Intern. Med.* 98 (1983): 284.

   J. L. Elliott, W. L. Hoopes, M. S. Platt et al., "The acquired immunodeficiency syndrome and *Mycobacterium avium-intracellulare* bacteremia in a patient with hemophilia," *Ann. Intern. Med.* 98 (1983): 290.

3. V. Fainstein, R. Bolivar, G. Mavligit et al., "Disseminated infection due to *Mycobacterium avium-intracellulare* in a homosexual man with Kaposi's sarcoma," *J. Infect. Dis.* 145 (1982): 586.

4. Davis, "Acquired immunodeficiency syndrome in a patient with hemophilia."

5. G. P. Wormser, L. B. Krupp, J. P. Hanrahan et al., "Acquired immunodeficiency syndrome in male prisoners," *Ann. Intern. Med.* 98 (1983): 297.

A. E. Pitchenik, M. A. Fischl, G. M. Dickinson et al., "Opportunistic infections and Kaposi's sarcoma among Haitians: evidence of a new acquired immunodeficiency state," *Ann. Intern Med.* 98 (1983): 277.

6. R. D. Diamond and C. C. Haudenschild, "Monocyte-mediated serum-independent damage to hyphal and pseudohyphal forms of *Candida albicans* in vitro," *J. Clin. Invest.* 67 (1981): 173.

7. D. Mildvan, "Opportunistic infections."

8. Ibid.
   Masur, "An outbreak."
   Pitchenik, "Opportunistic infections and Kaposi's sarcoma."
   J. Vieira, E. Frank, T. J. Spira et al., "Acquired immune deficiency in Haitians," *N. Engl. J. Med.* 308 (1983): 125.

9. Poon, "Acquired immunodeficiency syndrome with *Pneumocystis carinii*."
   Masur, "An outbreak."
   Masur, "Opportunistic infections in women."
   Fainstein, "Disseminated infection."
   Wormser, "Acquired immunodeficiency syndrome in prisoners."
   P. Zakowski, S. Fligiel, G. W. Berlin et al., "Disseminated *Mycobacterium avium-intracellulare* infection in homosexual men dying of acquired immunodeficiency," *JAMA* 248 (1982): 2980.
   J. B. Greene, G. S. Sidhu, S. Lewin et al., "*Mycobacterium avium-intracellulare*: a cause of disseminated life-threatening infection in homosexuals and drug abusers," *Ann. Intern. Med.* 97 (1982): 539.

10. R. H. Gentry, W. E. Farrar, Jr., T. A. Mahvi et al. "Simultaneous infection of the central nervous system with *Cryptococcus neoformans* and *Mycobacterium avium-intracellulare*," *South. Med. J.* 70 (1977): 865.

11. Greene, "*Mycobacterium avium-intracellulare*."

12. Poon, "Acquired immunodeficiency syndrome with *Pneumocystis carinii*."

13. Vieira, "Acquired immune deficiency in Haitians."

14. Pitchenik, "Opportunistic infections and Kaposi's sarcoma."

15. Ibid.
    A. E. Pitchenik, B. W. Russell, T. Cleary et al. "The prevalence of tuberculosis and drug resistance among Haitians," *N. Engl. J. Med.* 307 (1982): 162.

16. J. A. Krick and J. S. Remington, "Resistance to infection with *Nocardia asteroides*," *J. Infect. Dis.* 131 (1975): 665.

17. G. A. Filice, B. L. Beaman, J. A. Krick et al., "Effects of human neutrophils and monocytes on *Nocardia asteroides*. Failure of killing despite occurrence of oxidative metabolic burst," *J. Infect. Dis.* 142 (1980): 432.

18. C. A. Kaufman, K. S. Israel, J. W. Smith et al., "Histoplasmosis in immunosuppressed patients," *Am. J. Med.* 64 (1978): 923.
    S. C. Deresinski and D. A. Stevens, "Coccidioidomycosis in compromised hosts," *Medicine* 54 (1975): 277.

19. R. D. Diamond, "Inhibition of monocyte-mediated damage to fungal hyphae by steroid hormones," *J. Infect. Dis.* 147 (1983): 160.

20. J. Oleske, A. Minnefor, R. Cooper, Jr., et al., "Acquired immune deficiency syndrome in children," *JAMA* in press.

21. Pitchenik, "Opportunistic infections and Kaposi's sarcoma."

22. D. Lintz, R. Kapila, E. Pilgrim et al., "Nosocomial salmonella epidemic." *Arch. Int. Med.* 136 (1976): 968.

170 : NOTES AND SOURCES

23. P. Sen, J. K. Smith, M. Buse et al., "Modification of an experimental mouse Candida infection by human dialyzable leukocyte extract," *Sabouraudia* 20 (1982): 85.
24. Elliott, "Acquired immunodeficiency syndrome and *Mycobacterium*."
    Greene, "*Mycobacterium avium-intracellulare*."
25. D. K. Law, S. J. Dudrick, and N. I. Abdou, "Immunocompetence with protein-calorie malnutrition: the effects of nutritional repletion," *Ann. Intern. Med.* 79 (1973): 545.

    J. M. Oleske, M. L. Westphal, S. Shore et al., "Zinc therapy of depressed cellular immunity in acrodermatitis enteropathica," *Am. J. Dis. Child* 133 (1979): 915.

    A. E. Axelrod, "Nutrition in relation to immunity," in *Modern Nutrition—Health and Disease*, 6th edition, R. S. Goodheart and M. E. Schils, eds. (Philadelphia: Lea & Feboger, 1980), chapter 18, pp. 578–591.
26. Pitchenik, "Opportunistic infections and Kaposi's sarcoma."
27. Siegal, "Severe acquired immunodeficiency."
    Pitchenik, "Opportunistic infections and Kaposi's sarcoma."
28. Gentry, "Simultaneous infection."

Chapter 8. Kaposi's Sarcoma

SOURCES

DiGiovanna, J., and Safai, B. "Kaposi's sarcoma: retrospective study of 90 cases with particular emphasis on the familial occurrence, ethnic background and prevalence of other diseases." *Am. J. Med.* 71 (1981): 779–783.

Friedman-Kien, A. E. "Disseminated Kaposi's sarcoma syndrome in young homosexual men." *J. Am. Acad. Dermatol.* 5 (1981): 468–71.

Giraldo, G., Beth, E., and Haguenau, F. "Herpes-type virus particles in tissue culture of Kaposi's sarcoma from different geographic regions." *J. Natl. Cancer Inst.* 49 (1972): 1509–1526.

Giraldo, G., Beth, E., Kaurilsky, F., et al. "Antibody patterns to herpes viruses in Kaposi's sarcoma: serological association of European Kaposi's sarcoma with cytomegalovirus." *Int. J. Cancer* 15 (1975): 839–848.

Giraldo, G., Beth, E., Henle, W., et al. "Antibody patterns to herpes viruses in Kaposi's sarcoma. II. Serological associations of American Kaposi's sarcoma with cytomegalovirus." *Int. J. Cancer* 22 (1978): 126–131.

Giraldo, G., Beth, E., and Huang, E.-S. "Kaposi's sarcoma and its relationship to cytomegalovirus (CMV). III. CMV DNA and CMV early antigens in Kaposi's sarcoma." *Int. J. Cancer* 26 (1980): 23–29.

Harwood, A., Osoba, D., Hofstader, S., et al. "Kaposi's sarcoma in recipients of renal transplants." *Am. J. Med.*, 67 (1979): 759–765.

Kapadin, S., and Krause, J. "Kaposi's sarcoma after long-term alkylating agent therapy for multiple myeloma." *South. Med. J.* 70 (1977): 1011–1013.

Kaposi, M. "Idiopathisches multiples pigmentsarkom der haut." *Arch. Dermatol. Syphilol.* 4 (1872): 265–273.

Leung, F., Fam, A., and Osoba, D. "Kaposi's sarcoma complicating corticosteroid therapy for temporal artentis." *Am. J. Med.* 71 (1981): 320–322.

Myers, B., Kessler, E., Lepi, J., et al. "Kaposi's sarcoma in kidney transplant recipients." *Arch. Intern. Med.* 133 (1974): 307–311.

Nisce, L., Safai, B., and Poussin-Rosillo, H. "Once-weekly total and subtotal electron beam therapy for Kaposi's sarcoma." *CA* 47 (1981): 640–644.

Palmer, P. "Haemangiosarcoma of Kaposi." *Acta. Radiol.* (suppl) 316 (1972).

Pollack, M. S., Safai, B., Myskowski, P. L., et al. "Frequencies of HLA and GM immunogenetic markers in Kaposi's sarcoma tissue antigens" (submitted).

Reynolds, W., Winklemann, R., and Soule, E. "Kaposi's sarcoma: a clinicopathological study with particular reference to its relationship to the reticuloendothelial system." *Medicine* (Baltimore) 44 (1965): 419–443.

Safai, B., and Good, R. "Kaposi's sarcoma: a review and recent developments." *CA* 31 (1981): 2–12.

Safai, B., Miké, V., Giraldo, G., et al. "Association of Kaposi's sarcoma with second primary malignancies." *CA* 45 (1980): 1472–1479.

Taylor, J., Templeton, A., Vogel, C., et al.: "Kaposi's sarcoma in Uganda: a clinicopathological study." *Int. J. Cancer* 8 (1971): 122–135.

Taylor, J., and Ziegler, J. "Delayed cutaneous hypersensitivity reactions in patients with Kaposi's sarcoma." *Br. J. Cancer* 30 (1974): 312–318.

Templeton, A., and Hutt, M. "Distribution of tumors in Uganda." *Recent Results in Cancer Research* 41 (1973):1–22.

Urmacher, C., Myskowski, P., Ochoa, M., et al. "Outbreak of Kaposi's sarcoma in young homosexual men." *Am. J. Med.* 72 (1982): 569–575.

Vogel, C. L., Clements, D., Wanume, A. K., et al. "Phase II Clinical trials of BCNU (NSC409962) and bleomycin (NSC125066) in the treatment of Kaposi's sarcoma." *Cancer Chemother. Rep.* 57 (1973): 325–333.

Chapter 9. The Blood Bank Crisis

NOTES
1. Christine Russell, "Mysterious lethal disease spreads in U.S., government health officials fearful the pace is accelerating," *Washington Post*, Feb. 7, 1983.

   "Washington, D.C., news: Congress scrapes up $2,000,000 for AIDS," *Med. World News*, Jan. 24, 1983.
2. "Concerns on hepatitis B vaccine addresses," *Amer. Med. News*, Jan. 21, 1983.
3. Ibid.
4. Ibid.

   Michael Walzholz, "U.S. scientists doubt link between AIDS, hepatitis vaccine," *Wall Street Journal*, Feb. 11, 1983.
5. Walzholz, "U.S. scientists doubt link."
6. M. M. Leberman, O. D. Ratnoff, J. J. Scillian et al., "Impaired cell-mediated immunity in patients with classic hemophilia," *N. Engl. J. Med.* (1983): 79.
7. K. C. Davis, C. R. Horsburgh, U. Hasiba et al., "Acquired immunodeficiency syndrome in a patient with hemophilia," *Ann. Intern. Med.* 3 (1983): 284–286.

   M. Poon, A. Landay, E. F. Prasthofer et al., "Acquired immunodeficiency syndrome with *Pneumocystis carinii* pneumonia and *Mycobacterium avium-intra-*

cellulare infection in a previously healthy patient with classic hemophilia," *Ann. Intern. Med.* 98 (1983):287–290.

J. L. Elliott, W. L. Hoopes, M. S. Platt et al., "The acquired immunodeficiency syndrome and *Mycobacterium avium-intracellulare* bacteremia in a patient with hemophilia," *Ann. Intern. Med.* 98 (1983): 290–293.

8. Fackelheim, Kathy, "Search for AIDS agent intensified," *Clinical Chemistry News,* Feb. 1983, Vol. 9, No. 2.

9. Ibid.

10. J. B. Brunet et al., "Acquired immunodeficiency syndrome in France," *Lancet* 1 (1983): 700–701.

11. Fackelheim, "Search for AIDS."

12. J. Vieira, E. Frank, T. J. Spira et al., "Acquired immune deficiency in Haitians," *N. Engl. J. Med.* 308 (1983): 125.

Susan West, "One step behind a killer," *Science 83* (March 1983): 36.

13. West, "One step."

J. H. Joncas et al., "Acquired (or congenital) immunodeficiency syndrome in infants born of Haitian mothers," *N. Engl. J. Med.* 308 (1983): 842.

14. J. L. Marx, "Health officials seek ways to halt AIDS," *Science* 219 (1983): 271.

Chapter 10. Protecting Health Personnel

NOTES

1. S. M. Glick, "Humanistic medicine in a modern age," *N. Engl. J. Med.* 304 (1981): 1036.

2. J. Wyngaarden, *Cecil Textbook of Medicine* (Philadelphia: W. B. Saunders & Co., 1979).

3. L. Thomas, *Cecil Textbook of Medicine.*

4. Albert and Condie, "Handwashing patterns in intensive care units," *N. Engl. J. Med.* 304 (1981): 1465.

5. Michael Gottlieb, M.D., personal communication.

6. Merle Sande, M.D., personal communication.

Chapter 11. The Search for the Cause

NOTES

1. Centers for Disease Control, "A cluster of Kaposi's sarcoma and *Pneumocystis carinii* among homosexual male residents of Los Angeles and Orange Counties, California," *Morbidity and Mortality Weekly Report* 31 (1982): 305–307.

2. D. P. Francis, J. E. Maynard, "Transmission and outcome of hepatitis A, B, and non-A, non-B: a review," *Epidemiologic Rev.* 1 (1979): 17–31.

3. WHO International Study Teams, "Ebola haemorrhagic fever in Sudan, 1976," *Bull. WHO* 56 (1978): 247–270.

4. G. Offenstadt, P. Pinta, P. Hericord et al., "Multiple opportunistic infection due to AIDS in a previously healthy black woman from Zaire." *N. Engl. J. Med.* 308 (1983): 775.

Chapter 12. Where Do We Go from Here?

NOTES

1. Thucydides, *History of the Peloponnesian War*, translated by Rex Warner (New York: Penguin, 1954).
2. Barbara Tuchman, *Distant Mirror: The Calamitous 14th Century* (New York: Knopf, 1978).
3. Alfred W. Crosby, Jr., *Epidemic and Peace, 1918* (Westport, Conn.: Greenwood Press, 1976).
4. Allen C. Steere, Robert L. Grodzidki, Arnold N. Kornblatt et al., "The spirochetal etiology of Lyme disease," *N. Engl. J. Med.* 308 (1983): 733.
5. *Kuru, Early letters and field-notes from the Collection of D. Carleton Gajdusek,* Judith Farquhar and D. Carleton Gadjdusek, eds. (New York: Raven Press, 1981).
6. Mario Rizzetto, John L. Gerin, and Robert H. Purcell, "Delta antigen: evidence for a variant of hepatitis B virus or a non-A, non-B hepatitis agent," in *Perspectives in Virology XI,* (New York: Alan R. Liss, 1981).
7. Donald S. Fredrickson, " 'Venice' is not sinking (the water is rising): some views on biomedical research," *J. Amer. Med. Ass.* 247 (1982): 3072.

About the Authors

DONALD ARMSTRONG, M.D., is Chief, Infectious Disease Service, Director, Microbiology Laboratory, and Associate Chairman, Department of Medicine, Memorial Sloan-Kettering Cancer Center, New York; Professor of Medicine, Cornell University Medical College.

KEVIN M. CAHILL, M.D., is the Senior Member of the New York City Board of Health; Director, The Tropical Disease Center, Lenox Hill Hospital, New York; Clinical Professor of Public Health and Preventive Medicine, University of New Jersey—New Jersey Medical School, Newark; Professor and Chairman, Department of International Health, The Royal College of Surgeons, Ireland.

R. BEN DAWSON, M.D., is Director, Blood Transfusion Services and Research Laboratories, Professor of Pathology, University of Maryland School of Medicine and Hospital; Member of World Health Organization Expert Panel on Blood and Blood Products; formerly chairman of numerous national committees of the American Association of Blood Banks and the American Red Cross.

SYDNEY M. FINEGOLD, M.D., is Chief, Infectious Disease Section, Veterans Administration Wadsworth Medical Center; Professor of Medicine, UCLA School of Medicine, Los Angeles; immediate past president, Infectious Disease Society of America.

WILLIAM H. FOEGE, M.D., is Director, Centers for Disease Control, Public Health Service, U.S. Department of Health and Human Resources, Atlanta.

DONALD P. FRANCIS, M.D., is Chief Co-ordinator, AIDS Laboratory Activities, Center for Infectious Diseases, Centers for Disease Control, Public Health Service, U.S. Department of Health and Human Resources; formerly chief, World Health Organization Smallpox Program, U.P. India and Sudan.

DONALD S. FREDRICKSON, M.D., is Vice-President, Howard Hughes Medical Institute; formerly director, National Institute of Health, and scholar-in-residence, National Institute of Medicine.

ROBERT A. GOOD, M.D., Ph.D., is Member and Head, Cancer Research and Clinical Immunology Programs, Oklahoma Medical Research Foundation, Oklahoma City; Professor of Pediatrics, Research Professor of Medicine, and OMRF Professor of Microbiology and Immunology, University of Oklahoma Health Sciences Center; formerly president and scientific director, Memorial Sloan-Kettering Cancer Center.

SHELDON H. LANDESMAN, M.D., is Director, Antibiotic Laboratory, Director, Haitian AIDS Study Group, Downstate Medical Center, New York.

DONALD B. LOURIA, M.D., is Professor and Chairman, Department of Preventive Medicine and Community Health, University of New Jersey—New Jersey Medical School, Newark.

BIJAN SAFAI, M.D., is Chief, Dermatology Service, Memorial Sloan-Kettering Cancer Center; Associate Professor of Medicine, Cornell University Medical College; and Adjunct Member, The Rockefeller University.

DAVID J. SENCER, M.D., is Commissioner of Health, New York City; formerly director, Centers for Disease Control, Public Health Service, U.S. Department of Health and Human Services.

THEODORE WEISS, M.C., represents New York's 17th Congressional District in the U.S. House of Representatives. He is Chairman of the Government Operations Subcommittee on Intergovernmental Relations and Human Resources and is a Member of the Foreign Affairs Committee and the Select Committee on Children, Youth, and Families.

2659